Living Healthier Longer

with Dr. Ken Kroll

Restoring A Youthful You!
21st Century Science For Life

Kenneth M. Kroll M.D.

**Living Healthier Longer
With Dr. Ken Kroll**

ISBN: 1503303039
ISBN 13: 9781503303034
Library of Congress Control Number: 2014921001
CreateSpace Independent Publishing Platform
North Charleston, South Carolina

Dedicated to my always smiling,
always wonderful wife, Diane.
And to all you who want to avoid the "downsides," so
you can fully celebrate the "upside of life."

Introduction

This small book is about something quite personal, "the prolongation of healthy human life," and those things necessary to achieve it.

Now there are thousands of health and diet books, most so long and detailed (350 or more pages) you're unlikely to finish them or apply their myriad of information. The internet too has spawned additional millions of health-related sites and you-tube self-promotions, many pushing some "new breakthrough product you need to buy now."

This is a time when medical knowledge doubles every five years, and there are thousands of self-proclaimed healers and self-promoters – whether college professors, spa directors, or TV "health experts" selling their wares.

How is one to sort through this endless cacophony of confusion, conflict, chaos and misinformation? Even famous clinics get into the mix, promoting their own production of "white papers" and self-help books so we can better understand our breasts, our brains, or our prostate glands. And then there are well-meaning TV news channels hosting weekly medical "chiefs" expounding on a just released scientific study about some new drug, disease or threat to health – opinions that might change next month when the next "new study" is released.

And through all this fog – comes your "dark-cloud" neighbor who announces that this stuff is all bunk, that anyone sterilizing every door knob, and carefully measuring their alfalfa sprouts on their way to the gym every day so they can add 40 years to their life – will probably get hit by a Mack truck while crossing the street next week – and that enjoying life with shakes, fries, Fritos and hot fudge sundaes is the only way to enjoy life.

Even among well-trained physicians – the young doctor starting practice has learned the latest procedures and pharmaceuticals – but has little experience with any of them, and usually lacks the wisdom to know when things might be more hurtful than helpful. Forty years in practice studying patients, their diseases and treatments has given me a perspective – and hopefully a wisdom not present when I was younger - that are shared in this book.

If "The Art of Practicing Medicine (as defined by one of my Harvard instructors) is the ability to provide an adequate treatment based on inadequate evidence" – then *experience* becomes an indispensable ingredient to helping – and not harming a patient – or putting him or her thru an array of unnecessary tests, prescribed drugs or surgeries. Hopefully, *my 40 years experience* with medical practice and longevity science will make your pursuit of healthy life a much more successful one.

My medical-school training was basically to do two things: diagnose the correct disease, and then to dispense the right drug (or surgery when needed). My fifty-year journey as a physician-researcher-practitioner has changed many of my ideas on diagnosis and treatment – especially with reference to pharmaceuticals. So let me say just a word about drugs.

Drugs are synthetic, single-chemical compounds which block designated enzymatic and metabolic pathways in order to reduce a substance (e.g. cholesterol), a physiologic process (e.g. inflammation), or a symptom (e.g. pain). All drugs are unnatural substances in the human body, and all are, in various ways, toxic to human cell function. We call these toxicities "side effects." But all drugs can be lethal – as evidenced regularly on TV reports of deaths of young, famous personages – whether Michael Jackson, Anna Nicole Smith, Billy Mays – and dozens more – often in their 30s or 40s.

So – back to why this short book is being written. For just one reason: to give you the readers an experienced vision through the "fog" to settle on the few <u>Basics</u> upon which all true health is based, and a list of established power nutrients for you to consider. Included also is a brief tribute to those "natural health" pioneers who have made "natural" health and the American nutritional supplement market unique in all the world. In nutritional science, there's a whole new world unfolding that offers human health a support never before seen.

Simply put, this book is written to provide you the necessary tools to fashion your own personal life-enhancing anti-aging program.

And finally I've included bios of a couple recent "Giants of Science" that have made inspiring contributions to our long human struggle to relieve suffering, and Live Healthier Longer.

This book is written also as a tribute to Loren Israelson, esq. (Salt Lake City), Executive Director of the United Natural Products Alliance, and to Senator Orrin Hatch (R – Utah), Senator Tom Harkin (D – Iowa), and their staffs who drafted and fought so hard for passage of the very important DSHEA (Dietary Supplement and Health Education Act) – passed in 1994. Without DSHEA to constrain zealous FDA and Big Pharma anti-supplement activities, this book could not have been written.

Table of Contents

One

What Is Good Health?

A traditional formula for health would go something like this: "Eat a balanced diet, get a little exercise, and get a regular nights sleep." And what about sweets? You ask. The answer: "Desserts and sweets are fine, as long as you don't overdo it. In fact, a little sugar is good for you. And with a little exercise, you burn it off, anyways."

Sadly, this view is terribly off base. This may have worked a century ago when we lived on the family farm, raised our own fresh vegetables, butchered our own beef, pork, and chickens – and worked in the fields all day. But life today brings us a very different venue.

Today's world, for most of us, is a fast-paced, high-stress, punch-clock mixture of anxiety-producing uncertainties – job, school, careers, children, divorce, television news, high crime, pornography, violent movies, confused sexuality, fatigue, overweight, difficult finances, frustrating four-deep telephone menus, computer viruses, untrustworthy relationships, transient residences, increasingly complex "smart phones," TV violence with endless commercials, and drug ads that keep you wondering with their list of serious "side effects."

Dependable pillars like family, longtime friends, mainline churches, and reverence for God in schools have all come under attack from "progressive" forces – and predictably – violence, crime, divorce, teen-pregnancy rates, and homicides have all mushroomed, while psychiatrists and sociologists try to figure out what's causing this.

But putting aside the emotional and spiritual "stresses" that we endure, what are the *physical* stresses we bear in modern life. Let me list just a few:

⇒ Air polluted with toxic diesel truck fumes, auto and factory emissions

⇒ Toxic volatile organic chemicals (VOCs) off-gassing from synthetic carpets, paints, chipboard building materials, anti-fungal-fire-retardant chemicals on ceiling board, fabrics, plastics, furniture and new-car interiors.

⇒ Toxic water chemicals, from chlorine, lead, copper, or plastics from bottles we carry around

⇒ Fruits and vegetables containing fungicides, pesticides, and herbicide "weed killers."

⇒ Fresh meats containing antibiotics, hormones, or numerous other toxic chemicals from contaminated commercial animal feeds

⇒ Sausages and sandwich meats with toxic preservatives which produce carcinogenic nitrosamines in the human intestine

⇒ Highly-sugared soda pop, "sports" drinks and artificial "fruit drinks" that accelerate weight gain and aging. Diet sodas are even worse

⇒ White flour breads, pastries, donuts, muffins and cookies – virtually devoid of the vitamins, minerals, and phytonutrients found in organic whole grain wheat or oats.

⇒ Widespread use of artificial coloring agents – blue, red, yellow – found in candies, ice creams, breakfast cereals, sports drinks, and baked goods. These may contain small, but significant amounts of toxic heavy metals

⇒ Fish – most large ocean fish now contain toxic amounts of mercury and other toxins

⇒ Pharmaceutical drugs – all are toxic to human cell function

⇒ Virtually all packaged and processed foods sold on supermarket shelves: food coloring, preservatives, chemicals, or plasticizers (boxes, bags, cans, bottles)

In a sentence, we face multiple stresses, multiple toxicities, and multiple nutritional deficiencies virtually unknown to our ancestors – factors that make the traditional health advice inadequate and unworkable.

So, how then do we achieve good health within this new environment? An environment which is accelerating a wide range of chronic illnesses – from obesity to diabetes to cardiovascular disease to cancer to auto-immune disorders to ADD-ADHD and Autism to senile dementias. That is the challenge we face!! But fortunately, for those who value life and who treasure good health, there are real and effective remedies.

Let's lay out a simple, common-sense approach that can <u>maintain wellness</u> and <u>prevent disease</u> – issues which are essentially outside the practice of Western medicine. The well-trained M.D. is well-equipped to diagnose a disease after it has occurred, but offers almost nothing to prevent the disease, or to address the underlying cause of the disease. He or she practices Disease and Drug, not Prevention and Wellness.

We might more accurately call our present system "Sickness Care" rather than "Health Care."

Being a traditionally-trained M.D., I have great respect for the vaccines, the antibiotics, the anesthetic agents and some other meds which have saved millions and millions of lives. But, despite spending two or three times more per capita for health care than any other nation, the U.S. is 38th down the list for <u>longevity</u>! Something is clearly wrong and Americans clearly use far, far too many toxic drugs, and give too little attention to health-enhancing lifestyles, healthy eating and health-maintaining supplements!

In simplest terms, wellness, and long life depend on:

1. Changing the foods we eat, from processed, packaged, sugared, deep-fat fried and salted – to fresh, unprocessed, unboxed, unsugared, and minimally salted (i.e.: organic fresh fruit and fresh vegetables, grass-fed fresh meats, olive oil, fresh organic dairy, raw nuts, and organic whole grains). Because of GMO "hybrid" effects in grains, some people do better without wheat, or gluten in their diets. Avoid all corn, corn products, and all high-fructose corn syrup in food and drinks. New studies are showing that low-carb, medium "organic" fat, and medium animal-protein diets may be best. And

vegetarian-vegan diets, <u>though not part of our paleolithic past</u>, may have a place in helping manage certain severe disease states (e.g.: advanced atherosclerosis).

2. Reducing our fast-paced and toxic stresses, and finding time for emotional and spiritual growth.

3. Modest regular exercise; just walking a mile a day can do wonders; brief resistance exercise can build muscle.

4. Regular restful sleep 7 to 8 hours on a regular schedule. Forget TV violence and evening news shows; consider a book, a religious text, a meditation to enhance peace and purpose in the couple hours before retiring.

5. Add a few carefully chosen supplements. There are 30,000 out there. Many are over hyped, over priced and some even toxic. There are no "magic bullets" or single magic fruits. (See my list of basic key longevity supplements in Chapter 16)

6. Try to avoid prescription and over-the-counter drugs, unless they are life-saving, or used for a short course to manage an acute illness.

7. Avoid toxins whenever you can – food colorings, most preservatives, thickeners, conditioners, flavor enhancers (MSG), partially hydrogenated trans-fats, high fructose corn syrup in drinks and breads, mercury-laced fish, tobacco, excess alcohol, and excess caffeine. Avoid all energy drinks and all soda pop! And no, ice cream is not a health food. Read the ingredients.

8. Maintain good intestinal health with daily plain, unsugared organic yogurt and/or Kefir.

Follow these reasonably simple guidelines; you'll add healthy years and length to your life.

A word of caution: The marketplace is full of exotic "super fruit" juices and "unique substances" guaranteed from the Garden of Eden, a tropical oasis, a cave from Bill Bill Bomba, or a deep hole in the Gobi Dessert. Sadly, most of their cure-all health claims stretch the truth. Now I don't mean to make fun of good companies doing an honest job with helpful products, but I've watched the natural products industry for many years and companies understandably want to make every claim possible to sell products. But much of this is folklore-based, with unproven exaggerated claims and has shaky mouse science behind it.

Trustworthy sources of raw materials, methods of extraction, effective amounts, and well-planned human clinical trials must all be considerations for a legitimate health product. For any single vitamin, mineral, herb or tropical fruit juice to claim it has all the answers for good health is simply misinformation. Even the best scientists don't have all the answers, and today's panacea too often becomes tomorrow's detriment to health. Hype should not be mistaken for health.

So what's the body like when everything's working well, and we feel full of vitality physically and emotionally?

Allow me to compare a body in excellent health to a great worldwide symphony orchestra. Thousands of cornets, trumpets, French horns, tubas, saxophones, clarinets, oboes, bassoons, cellos, violas, violins, stringed basses, drums, cymbals, castanets, and harps – when working together on a single musical score – produce a harmonious melody that is balanced, pure, and satisfying. But let the horns not coordinate with the strings, or the percussion not coordinate with the woodwinds – and a dissonance develops that shatters our senses, or at the very least creates an uneasiness within us so we wonder what's wrong.

Similarly, the human body is an unbelievably complex symphony of activities – millions of biochemical processes influenced by hormones, vitamins, minerals, amino acids, fatty acids, polyphenols, food-derived plant nutrients (phytonutrients), communication molecules, neurotransmitters, transcription factors, second messengers, prostaglandin eicosanoids, and a vast array of other yet-unnamed molecules that will take many years to sort out.

And when any of these millions (yes, millions) of biochemical reactions are partly deranged by toxins, stress, or nutrient deficiencies – our human symphony continues on, but in abnormal ways that we finally recognize as a disease, fatigue, accelerated aging, or "just not feeling well."

So, the great question is: can well formulated and scientifically supported nutritional products help keep the complex human symphony harmonious?

My firm belief is an emphatic YES. And now there is powerful science and epidemiological evidence to support this YES. And while so many high-priced "exotic" juice drinks make exaggerated health claims, they probably offer little more health benefit than a small glass of fresh squeezed orange juice or a glass of organic concord grape juice! Sadly, by the time most exotic fruit juices have been squeezed, concentrated, dehydrated, preserved, processed, and pasteurized (things not listed on labels) most have much-reduced nutritional value and show no relation to the test tube or mouse studies done on specialized extracts of the fruit or berry.

While avoiding complex research models that employ "nodal network analysis" or "macromolecular crowding" in cell molecular biology, we must nonetheless rise above much of the simplistic single-molecule function analysis spawned by Western medicine's long-term affiliation with pharmaceutical drug research. Human cell function is infinitely more complicated than single-chemical (drug) therapies could likely address without significant toxic side effects.

Let's finish this chapter by asking, <u>What is Aging?</u> Addressing this long-pondered question has led to numerous theories of aging, several of which clearly play important roles – such as the free-radical theory, the Hayflick limit, or the telomere-shortening concept.

But in general terms, aging can be defined as the general breakdown of the metabolic processes essential to cell and organ survival. And in this context, any organ's failure can lead to death, and can be the weak link in our chain of life.

This common-sense view allows us to focus – for optimal health – on preserving those major organ systems expressing the major degenerative diseases – Cardiovascular System (heart attacks, strokes and peripheral arterial disease), Nervous System (Alzheimer's disease, Parkinson's disease, other neurodegenerative disorders), Metabolic-Hormonal System (overweight, obesity, diabetes, metabolic syndrome), Immune System (Infections, HIV, Cancer).

Preserving these organ systems is another way of understanding what this book is all about.

My goal is to help you really take personal responsibility for your own health with information that can
get you off the treadmill of doctor visits, toxic drugs,
toxic stress, and shortened life. Yes, you can control
your own healthy well-being and longevity! Read on!

Two

A Little History

For the forty-plus years I've watched the natural products marketplace turn into the ten-billion dollar industry we find today – growing up in Southern California as a surfer and bodybuilder – I've seen some remarkable breakthroughs, some exciting health products, and some amazing science come forward. The current generation is probably unfamiliar with gigantic scientific breakthroughs like the discovery of penicillin by Sir Alexander Fleming – (1928 - 1941), the discovery of a vaccine to prevent the terrible disease poliomyelitis (Dr. Jonas Salk – 1955) (*see sidebar 1*), or vaccines to prevent the terrible deaths from yellow fever or smallpox. To Americans today, these are "old history." Hospitals filled with large "iron lung" machines to keep paralyzed polio victims breathing are not part of current public consciousness.

But where did the idea of "health foods" and natural product wellness originate? In ancient times, as found in the Torah (Bible Old Testament) God instructed the Jews to eat certain foods and to avoid others. Thus was born the concept that food choices matter for health. In more modern times we witnessed an era of self-trained health gurus, some with sound health advice, others hucksters of harmful habits and nostrums. The realm of "health foods" blossomed with the discovery of vitamins in the early 1900s. This also began the era of promoters, potions, and magical panaceas. But many were devotees to wellness, healthy eating and making good lifestyle choices.

"Health food" pioneers included Adelle Davis ("Eat Right to Keep Fit," "Let's Have Happy Children"), Gaylord Hauser ("Diet Does It," "Be Happy, Be Healthier," "Mirror, Mirror On The Wall"), Victor Lindlahr ("You Are What You Eat"), Johanna Brandt ("The Grape Cure For Cancer"), Paul Bragg ("The Miracle of Fasting"), Jack LaLanne ("The Benefits of Juicing"), Harvey Diamond ("Fit For Life"), and John Robbins, ("Diet For a New America").

As nutritional science started to expand, a whole new generation of natural-product health experts has appeared. These include currently famous researchers like Barry Sears, PhD. ("Enter the Zone," "The Anti-Aging Zone"), Jeffrey Bland, PhD., ("20-Day Rejuvenation Diet Program" and founder of

The Institute of Functional Medicine), Robert Atkins, M.D., ("Dr. Atkins New Diet Revolution"), Michael Eades, M.D. ("The Protein Power Life Plan"), Andrew Weil, M.D. ("8 Weeks to Optimum Health"), Drs Richard and Rachael Heller ("The Carbohydrate Addicts Diet"), Walter Willett, M.D. ("Eat, Drink, and Be Healthy"), Arthur Agatson, M.D. ("The South Beach Diet"), Eric Braverman, M.D. ("Younger You") and dozens more. (Jean Carper, Richard Passwater, Abram Hoffer, Balz Frei, Candace Pert, Michael Murray, Bruce Ames, Jordan Rubin, Dr. John Lee, Anne Louise Gittleman, and Dr. Mark Hyman)

In this brief history I should mention seven other books that have brought major new insights into our understanding of human health: "Nutrition and Physical Degeneration" by Weston A. Price, DDS, "The Antioxidant Miracle" by Lester Packer, PhD., "Genetic Nutritioneering" by Jeffrey Bland, PhD., "The Paleo Answer" by Loren Cordain, PhD, "Ultra Metabolism" by Mark Hyman, M.D., "The Fast Diet" by Dr. Michael Mosley and "Grain Brain" by David Perlmutter, M.D. These authors have confirmed:

- the almost unfathomable complexity of the human body, human genetics, and psycho-neuro-endocrine-immuno-entero-enzymatic processes

- the supreme importance of natural foods and nutrients for cells and organs to optimally perform their complex activities

- a rational *holistic* basis for maintaining wellness and preventing disease

- a reasonable basis for reversing and even "curing" many diseases *without need for pharmaceuticals*

This last proposition will, of course, be the most controversial in a society so locked into traditional pharmaceutical approaches to medical treatment, entrenched unhealthful dietary habits, and high-stress sedentary lifestyles.

And since the Human Genome Project, completed in 2003 under the direction of Dr. Francis Collins, computer driven studies are starting to understand the genetic changes seen in disease development. (Francis Collins' book, "The Language of God," copyrighted 2006 has become a classic in support of belief in God and the Bible by one of the world's leading scientists.) *(see sidebar 2)*

This genetic approach to understanding human diseases is also revealing how food, nutrients, and supplements positively influence gene expression. Food substances cause "up-regulation" or "down regulation" of genes that cause important changes in cell and organ functions, and that determine wellness or sickness.

Do genetics therefore determine what diseases we will get and how long we will live?

A major misconception regarding longevity is that how long our parents lived will likely determine how long we will live and "we should pick our parents wisely." While genetics does, of course, play a role, current science supports a quite different view.

In their landmark 1998 study, (the MacArthur Foundation Study of Aging in America) Dr. John Rowe, M.D., and Dr. Robert Kahn, M.D., in their book "Successful Aging" – demonstrate that only about 30% of one's lifespan will be determined by heredity, and 60 – 70% will be determined by one's lifestyle choices.

There is now strong-evidence that good lifestyle choices can not only prevent most chronic degenerative diseases associated with aging, and can reverse many of those diseases after they've occurred, but remarkably, can significantly delay or ameliorate even familial, genetically-determined diseases.

Recognizing these new understandings, this book will, in a simple format, outline those lifestyle choices that "evidence-based" science shows can "make straight your path" to living healthier longer.

(And yes, I've read all the books listed in this chapter.)

Giants of Science (sidebar 1)

Jonas Salk, M.D., PhD (1914 – 1995), an American medical researcher and virologist, was born in New York City of uneducated Russian-Jewish immigrant parents. Early in his medical education, Salk decided against a private practice with its financial rewards, and to pursue only medical research.

And in 1947, at the University of Pittsburg, he encountered the National Foundation for Infantile Paralysis, and wondered if it would be possible to find an answer to the polio "plague" threatening the U.S. His earlier research with flu virus and flu vaccines had served as a foundation for his new interest in polio viruses.

Until 1955, when the Salk vaccine was introduced, polio was the most frightening disease in the U.S. Annual epidemics kept getting worse and victims were usually children. By 1952 there were 300,000 reported cases, and 58,000 deaths, mostly children. Citizens of big cities were terrified each summer as the "polio plague" returned. America's president FDR himself became a victim at age 39, never again to be without a wheelchair.

But polio proved a difficult challenge, and Salk worked long days and many nights for 8 years until it appeared he had a "killed virus" vaccine that might work. Fear of being injected with the polio virus, alive or dead, was so great that Salk had to first inject himself, his wife, and his three children to demonstrate the vaccine's safety. Then came a controversial large national trial with the unproven vaccine. On April 12, 1955 Dr. Thomas Francis, Jr. announced by radio "the vaccine is proving safe and effective with a 90% success rate." Church bells rang across the country, synagogues and churches held prayer meetings, and parents and teachers wept openly. Salk was heralded as a national hero, and millions around the world were inoculated. Polio cases dropped almost to zero, and today poliomyelitis is almost unknown. The death of so many children, the paralyzed bodies, the shriveled lifeless legs of children on crutches or in wheel chairs became only painful memories.

In 1965, in a 10th anniversary tribute to Jonas Salk and his vaccine, Luther Terry, Surgeon General of the United States proclaimed, "This represents an historic triumph of preventive medicine – unparalleled in human history."

Giants of Science (sidebar 2)

Frances S. Collins, M.D., PhD, is a physician-geneticist noted for his leadership of the Human Genome Project, a 15 year Herculean milestone completed in 2003. This epic event in human history resulted in Dr. Collins being awarded the Presidential Medal of Honor by President George W. Bush in 2007. And in 2009, he was nominated by President Barack Obama to become Director of the prestigious U.S. National Institutes of Health. Dr. Collins is one of the top scientists in the world, and his groundbreaking work has changed the very ways we consider our health and examine disease.

"I am truly honored and humbled to take the helm today (August 17, 2009) of the world's leading organization supporting biomedical research," Dr. Collins said. "The scientific opportunities in both the basic and clinical realms are unprecedented, and the talent and dedication of (NIH scientists and staff) guarantee that this will be a truly exciting era."

NIH has more than 19,000 employees, a fiscal 2014 budget of $31 billion, and supports more than 325,000 research personnel at more than 3,100 institutions throughout the U.S., and around the world.

Dr. Collins has had a longstanding interest in the interface between science and faith having himself journeyed from atheist to bible believer. His 2006 book

"The Language of God: A Scientist Presents Evidence For Belief" spent many weeks on the New York Times best seller list.

Three

Your Powerful
Microbiome

I f asked "what is our largest human interface (exposure) to the outside world?" – most people would re-
ply: "Our skin, of course." Unfortunately, this is not
even close to being correct.

The body's largest surface stretching 100 times
greater than our skin is the unfolded surface of the human intestine – enough to cover an entire tennis court!
This very large surface is exposed to the trillions of
bacteria, fungi, molds, viruses, parasites and poisons
everywhere around us! Yes, if all the villi, crypts and
folded surfaces within our 25 plus feet of intestine
were spread out flat, it would be this unbelievably
large surface.

But let's ask, what exactly does the intestine do, and how much influence does it have on our bodily processes?

If you are overweight, and have belly bulge, are fatigued, depressed or moody, crave sweets, always hungry and have poor sleep patterns, have gas, bloating and "stomach cramps," the odds are high that your microbiome is to blame.

And this is where recent science has been revealing a most astonishing story.

The tough keratin coating of skin cells protects it from millions of infectious intruders, allowing only the sun's ultra-violet rays to penetrate and convert cholesterol molecules to Vitamin D.

The gut lining, by contrast is engaged in a constant violent warfare with trillions of bacteria, and thousands of species of fungi, molds, yeasts, viruses, and dozens of diarrhea-producing food-poisoning "bugs"– some lethal.

What is your <u>microbiome</u>?

Your microbiome is the total mass of the trillions of non-human cellular organisms that inhabit your intestine – average weight about <u>three pounds</u> (same approximate weight as your brain).

This biome "alternate universe," we now know, exerts a powerful influence on every organ system in your body! It eats some of the foods you consume, produces vitamins, and controls your absorption of thousands of vitamins, minerals, trace minerals – and toxins – that arrive during digestion.

Your microbiome can be healthy and balanced, or can be unbalanced and negatively affect your health. Of the 500-plus bacterial species present there are trillions of "good" bacteria and trillions of "bad" bacteria that create a "shifting balance" between types that strengthen our health, and types that damage our health. And this "balance" is determined by the foods we eat, or even the antibiotics we use. Antibiotics kill off trillions of your good bacteria, and can create an unhealthy balance in your microbiome.

And since 70 – 80% of your immune system is located immediately surrounding the gut, your microbiome has a major affect on your immune system, an effect that is critical, since it's the immune system that must combat viruses, infections, and even cancer.

Aside from some help from stomach acid and pancreatic enzymes, it is your microbiome bacteria that "digest" your food, control your appetite, orchestrate your immune system, affect your mood, and have a controlling influence on even how your genes get expressed. **A more realistic way to understand all this is that we are each two co-equal universes working in symbiosis (i.e. working together).**

So we have not only our recently defined human genome, but also a second full genome within us – both operating to keep us alive.

The crucial question then is: How do we control these two powerful genomes? The answer to this question will determine everything about us – from mood, to weight, to disease, to how long we will live!

The answer remains: **"You are what you eat." What we eat determines the particular bacterial balance in your microbiome. And this in turn decides your state of body health, mental health, and longevity.**

Bottom line: follow the diet suggestions outlined in this book, and favor extra probiotics like plain, low-fat, unsweetened yogurt (Nancy's Organic plain low-fat or whole milk yogurt at Sprouts, Whole Foods, and other health food stores) and low fat unsweetened Kefir from many stores. Avoid "Greek" yogurts. And avoid antibiotics whenever you can, and never use long-term antibiotics.

If you feel your gut needs still more help, pick up a "used copy" of "The Microbiome Diet" by Raphael Kellman, M.D., at Amazon Books.

Four

The Benefits of Berries

"An overwhelming body of research has now firmly established that the dietary intake of berry fruits has a positive and profound impact on human health, performance, and disease."

N.P. Seeram, PhD., Assistant Director
Center for Human Nutrition
University of California at Los Angeles
J.Agric.FoodChem.2008,26,627- 629

During the past ten or twenty years, there has been an exciting new interest in the health benefits – not only of fruits and vegetables in general – but of berries in particular. Research scientists have demonstrated that polyphenols in berries are not only antioxidants that neutralize free-radicals, but may also prevent age-related memory loss and diseases like Parkinson's and Alzheimer's. Such benefits come not only from effects on free-radicals, but from the way cells "talk" to one another (e.g. neuro-endocrine communication, and stress signal transduction). [1]

These positive effects on brain function include not only things like memory, concentration, focus, and creative thinking – but also motor functions that control walking, sense of balance and other physical activities. [2, 3]

But there's another factor that plays into this equation of how healthy a berry or a fruit is for us. It has to do with how much stress or struggle the berry or fruit encounters for its own survival – survival against viruses, fungi, ultra-violet radiation, plant diseases, and insect predators – to name a few. In other words, the fruit or plant has its own "immune system." The interesting health principle here is that those fruits that have survived in the most challenging environments, have developed the more robust immune system substances or phyto (plant) nutrients. And to carry this a step further, it appears that those fruits surviving in these challenging environments, are those with the richest nutrients to benefit human health, and increase our abilities to survive the health challenges and diseases *we* face. Berries grown wild, and those from extreme weather areas like the arctic, usually have the best ratings for health benefits.

So then we have to ask, are there ways to measure the amount of these protective nutrients in our fruits, vegetables, and foods? The answer is – yes. And while these test-tube methods don't automatically translate into human health benefits, they are very useful ways to preview likely health benefits. And more importantly, at our present level of scientific understanding, *these tests do seem to equate fairly well with how beneficial a food will be to human health.*

Currently, one of the more useful of these tests is called the ORAC test (Oxygen Radical Absorbance Capacity). Dark colored berries all have high ORAC scores! A food's bioavailability as well as level of vitamins, minerals, trace minerals, amino acids, fatty acids and many other phytonutrients are additional issues, only in small part measured by ORAC scores. However, we now accept free-radical induced inflammation and oxidation as causative factors of virtually all chronic degenerative diseases (atherosclerosis, heart attacks, strokes, auto-immune disorders, neurodegenerative diseases like Parkinson's and Alzheimer's), - and of the aging process itself. The antioxidant, anti-inflammation and nutrient activities of foods are felt to be of vital importance to avoiding, and sometimes reversing, these diseases and enjoying longer, healthier life.

With America's aging population and the dramatic increase in Alzheimer's and other senile dementias the issue of prevention is a serious one. Keeping our focus on berries, the question arises whether berry nutrients, such as polyphenols, are adequately absorbed from the intestine to be beneficial. And if absorbed, can they cross the blood-brain barrier to be beneficial to brain cells?

A recent (2009) review of these issues by the Human Nutrition Center on Aging at Tufts University (Boston) concluded that not only are berry nutrients bioavailable (absorbed thru the intestine), but in fact "do accumulate in the brain following long-term consumption." They conclude further that "berry fruit supplementation has continued to demonstrate efficacy in reversing age-related cognitive decline in animal studies."[4]

A 2008 human study from the National Public Health Institute (Helsinki, Finland) tested HDL ("good" cholesterol), blood pressure, and platelet adhesion (e.g. tendency to form clots in coronary arteries) with subjects consuming a modest portion (3.5 ounces) of mixed berries a day for 8 weeks. HDL levels increased significantly, and systolic blood pressure decreased significantly in those with hypertension, and there was a significant decrease in platelet adhesiveness. The authors conclude that berries may be important dietary factors in the prevention of cardiovascular disease. [5]

Thus far in this chapter we've concluded that numerous in vitro and in vivo studies are showing that modest regular consumption of berries likely improves brain function, helps prevent senile dementias, supports healthy cardiovascular function, decreases high blood pressure, decreases tendency for clot formation as seen in heart attacks and strokes, raises HDL (good) cholesterol levels, and that berries are powerful non-toxic antioxidant and anti-inflammation substances. Other studies on berries suggest they play significant roles in preventing some cancers.

Virtually all berry researchers attribute these very significant health benefits primarily to the <u>Polyphenols</u> contained in berries. These phyto (plant) chemicals are present in virtually all fruits and vegetables – but are especially rich in berries.

Another important feature of dark-purple berries is their anthocyanins content. These are the pigments that give the berry its color. Anthocyanins are now believed to act not only as antioxidants, but also as beneficial genetic modulators, signaling healthy responses by "upregulating" one, two, thirty or a thousand different genes to provide a wide variety of responses in the ultra-complex "machinery" that regulates the life of the cell, or of a system (e.g. immune system), or of an organ (e.g. the liver or brain). We are still many years away from understanding the interplay between the thousands of nutrients contained in our foods – and the millions of metabolic, genetic, hormonal, and neurological processes influenced by those nutrients. But we can make an important observation at this point – namely – *that it is impossible for the human body to remain healthy when the foods we consume are devoid of the nutrients it requires for health.* Sadly, the over-processed, artificially colored, over-sugared, over-salted, nutrient-deficient foods that are "staples" of the American diet and that fill the shelves of our supermarkets will predictably lead to what we call "the chronic degenerative diseases of aging" – the overweight, the diabetes, heart attacks, strokes, autoimmune disorders, senile dementias, depression and mood disorders so prevalent today. And in our children, the epidemic of autism, ADD, ADHD, asthma, overweight, and violence also has roots in deficient diets of mother and child.

A good example of how these polyphenol substances translate into protection from disease can be tested by seeing if they inhibit LDL oxidation. LDL (the "bad" cholesterol) oxidation is the critical initial step to the development of atherosclerosis, which in turn results in heart attacks, strokes, hypertension, renal failure, and senile dementias. Berry anthocyanins have been shown to inhibit LDL oxidation. (9)

For us, the important issue is that polyphenols are powerful additions to our diet, that the actions of polyphenols go far beyond their role as antioxidants, and that berries are particularly rich sources of these health-giving substances. So, enjoy daily servings of blueberries, blackberries, acai berries, maqui berries, bilberries, loganberries strawberries, and boysenberries. And don't forget cranberries, cherries, pomegranate and black grapes – all rich in polyphenol nutrients. And, if you can find them, don't overlook arctic Scandinavian berries like lingonberries and golden cloudberries – both considered superfruits.

But let's move on now to a group of very important supplements I've selected as options you may add to your own personalized living healthier longer program.

Five

Power Nutrients

While lifestyle choices can account for about 70% of our living healthier longer success, we also know that human cells are extremely complex "factories" that require thousands of "raw materials" to function optimally. And on planet earth, these raw materials come from sun-stimulated plant life. And the health advantages that come from eating animal meats is simply that the "grass fed" animal has turned large amounts of plant life into quality protein, including a wide range of important fatty acids, vitamins, minerals, trace minerals and other nutritious factors. Thus animal meats, eggs and dairy represent pre-processed and concentrated plant-life nutrition, which save us from munching grass, lettuce, and leaves eight hours a day, as do many less advanced animal species.

In this book the previous chapter pointed out the unique benefits of eating berries. Now I've selected nine special power nutrients that are powerful promoters of disease-free living. A dozen or two others could be added, but these are my favorites for this book. These are not all required for your daily great-health program, but should be considered when you put together your own personal program as outlined in Chapter 17.

N-Acetyl Cysteine
Alpha Lipoic Acid
Green Tea and Green Tea Extract
Bocopa monnieri
Astaxanthin
Resveratrol
Grape Seed Extract
Curcumin
Adaptogens

These power nutrients are metabolic enhancers backed by thousands of scientific studies by some of the world's most distinguished PhD biochemists and research scientists. Plug each ingredient into PubMed or a dozen other databases and you'll find a wealth of research to document powerful health benefits.

Six

Power Nutrient – Glutathione

Let's start with a combination of the first two power ingredients – N-Acetyl Cysteine and Alpha Lipoic Acid. Each of these is a powerhouse unto itself with hundreds of scientific research studies supporting their health benefits. I could literally write a book about each, but for purposes of this book, we'll discuss them together, as substances that play important roles together in the production of <u>Glutathione.</u> So what is Glutathione?

Glutathione is the body's master wellness molecule! It is present in all cells and organs. In general terms Glutathione is the master <u>antioxidant</u> in the human body. Everyone knows, for example, that vitamin E is an important lipid-phase antioxidant. And indeed it is. But there are a million times more molecules of

Glutathione at work in each cell than there are molecules of vitamin E.

Glutathione is a tri-peptide, composed of three amino acids – glutamine, cysteine, and glycine. And Glutathione has many important functions beyond being the master antioxidant.

Virtually all human diseases are associated with low Glutathione levels (10) and Glutathione deficiency is now felt to play an active role in aging, age-related macular degeneration, diabetes, heart disease, cancer, inflammatory bowel disorders, Parkinson's disease, Alzheimer's, and neurodegenerative disorders – just to name a few. The science of Glutathione in human health and disease has become so important that a database search on PubMed (U.S. National Institutes of Health) displayed over 87,000 scientific research articles involving Glutathione!

Let's list a few of its most important activities:

- Glutathione protects the mitochondria (the "factories" that produce energy in all cells – energy for the cell to stay alive and do its work.) (11) It does this by preventing damage to the delicate lipid membranes that surround each mitochondrion, preventing damage to the DNA present in each mitochondrion, and preventing damage to the many enzymes operating within the mitochondria. It's worth noting that our most active cells – those using the most energy – are in brain, heart, liver, and kidneys – and most of these busy cells will have hundreds or thousands of mitochondria within each of them. Dr. Denham Harman, father of the free-radical theory of aging, and many other longevity scientists now feel that the principle cause of aging is free radical damage to mitochondria. (12)

• Glutathione plays a major role in detoxification. For that reason some of the highest intracellular levels of glutathione are present in liver cells, the liver being the place where most detoxification occurs.

• Glutathione plays a major role as a regenerator of other antioxidants like vitamin C, vitamin E, vitamin A, catalase, superoxide dismutase, and others.

• Glutathione chelates heavy metals and facilitates their removal from the body - metals like mercury, lead, aluminum, cadmium, arsenic and iron.

• Glutathione helps prevent AGEs (Advanced Glycation End Products), products that accelerate aging and disease production.

- Glutathione plays the major support role for the anti-infection, anti-cancer activities of the immune system.

One might now ask: If glutathione is so central and critical a substance for life, wellness, and longevity – why don't we all take glutathione pills daily?

Many companies, in fact, offer a glutathione oral supplement. However, the best scientific evidence indicates that taking glutathione by mouth might be of little value, since stomach acid hydrolyzes the molecule and breaks it down to its three amino acids, and intracellular glutathione levels are not always improved. Stated more simply, oral glutathione is not considered ideally bioavailable!

But good studies indicate unequivocally that ingestion of Glutathione precursors N-Acetyl Cysteine and Alpha Lipoic Acid are absorbed thru the intestine, enter cells and elevate intracellular glutathione rather dramatically. One of the first research biochemists to demonstrate this precursor effect was Lester Packer, PhD from University of California at Berkeley. He describes this important research in his breakthrough book, "The Antioxidant Miracle" published by John Wiley and Sons in 1999. (Lester Packer is regarded as one of the world's foremost antioxidant research scientists.)

Seven

Power Nutrient – Green Tea

W e turn now to a substance first found in China around 2700 B.C. by Emperor Shen Nung, well before the advent of the Tang and Sung Dynasties. But it was from the Tang Dynasty that the world's first great treatise on tea (ch'a) came from LuYu. His comprehensive work reigned supreme for five hundred years and LuYu has aptly been labeled "the Patron Saint of Tea."

Today more tea is drunk worldwide than any other beverage except water. (13) From China to England, from India to Tibet, from Marseilles to Murmansk it is relished as a beverage of choice. Each day over one and a half billion cups of tea are consumed on the planet. Perhaps no other beverage has been the object of such sanctification and rituals. All the beauty of the Japanese way of life is embodied in its tea ceremony. And "tea time" in Britain has dominated daily schedules for centuries. Devotees to a rich Assam, a delicate Darjeeling, or an aromatic Jasmine would be offended by the thick, black, bitter, and harsh bite that addicted coffee drinkers regularly endure. Even as a stimulant, tea is much gentler and much lower in caffeine than even a "gourmet" Arabica coffee. While coffee jangles the nerves and stresses the body, tea soothes the body while gently enhancing mental function.

For purposes of this discussion though, we want to turn our attention to the remarkable health benefits that put tea in a class by itself. While green or black tea both provide health benefits, it appears that green tea has a slight edge.

While tea is a botanical with over a hundred phytochemicals in its makeup – including minerals, trace minerals, amino acids and other nutrients, the most studied nutrient is EGCG (epigallocatechin gallate).

Polyphenols such as flavonols, flavandiols, flavonoids, and phenolic acids are abundant in green tea. Among the flavonols, the catechins are of special interest and are responsible for many of the impressive health benefits found in tea.

So, what are some recognized benefits from green tea and EGCG?

- EGCG is over 200 times more powerful than vitamin E in neutralizing the lipid free radicals that can damage brain cells.

- A Korean study suggests that EGCG has protective effects against beta-amyloid induced brain-cell death, and "may be beneficial for the prevention of Alzheimer's disease." [14]

- An important 2006 Italian study in men showed green tea catechins were "very effective" at preventing cancer of the prostate in men who already had pre-cancerous changes by biopsy! [15]

- An important 2006 Japanese study in humans concluded that "green tea consumption is associated with reduced mortality due to all causes (including that due to cardiovascular disease)." [16]

- A 2005 U.S. human study (meta analysis) suggests that green tea may play a role in prevention of breast cancer, and may also help prevent metastatic disease. [17]

- Green tea seems to lessen joint degeneration in lab models of rheumatoid arthritis.

- Long term tea consumption showed significant improvements in bone-mineral density throughout the body including lumbar spine and hip regions. In other words, it helps prevent adult osteoporosis. [18]

- An important Dutch Study ("The Rotterdam Study") concluded that "an increased intake of tea and flavonoids may significantly prevent fatal myocardial infarction (heart attack)."[19]

- Green tea may help for weight loss since it can increase calorie and fat metabolism.

- Green tea exhibits anti-viral activity for some human viruses.

Thus, green tea has a long history supporting good health. While it is not a "magic bullet" or a cure all, it is an important addition to the diet.

My recommendation: Look for a Japanese green tea like Sencha – Japanese green teas have long been considered the highest quality available.

Eight

Power Nutrient –
Bacopa Monnieri

One of the most revered plant-herbs of ancient Ayervedic Medicine – one that has stood the test of time as a "brain tonic" is Bacopa Monnieri, otherwise known in India as Brahmi.

In modern India, Bacopa is used to treat Alzheimer's, senile dementias, epilepsy, attention deficit hyperactivity disorder (ADHD), anxiety disorders, panic attacks, and allergic conditions. Thus it is purported to be an antioxidant, anti-inflammatory, memory enhancer, and brain rebalancer. These are remarkable attributes for a non-toxic all natural plant extract! And modern scientific studies are starting to strongly support these claims. But before we list several of these seminal studies, let's briefly discuss "memory," and also Alzheimer's disease.

Memory is a complex phenomenon. When a new piece of knowledge first enters the brain, it's put into what we call short-term memory. Then thru a complex series of steps including the importance you attach to it, the rate of mindful repetition of the knowledge, and to what previous knowledge it relates – your brain moves it into long-term memory. This entire process requires millions of brain cells "talking with each other" through communication molecules called neurotransmitters. This, in turn, requires that the involved brain cells be healthy and their energy production unimpeded. Other factors can speed up or slow down this whole process. For example, lack of sleep, fatigue, anxiety, worry, and depression can slow the process. Good rest and being happy, hopeful, alert, focused, and motivated – all speed up the memory process.

Scientists now believe that Bacopa's proven ability to enhance memory probably means it positively modulates multiple brain functions. For example, reducing anxiety, calming the mind, neutralizing brain free-radicals, and increasing alertness would all help the learning and memory process. In these ways, it may even improve intelligence! I'll share some recent studies supporting all this in a minute.

But first let's briefly look at Alzheimer's disease. Alzheimer's we know damages short-term memory. It's not unusual in early Alzheimer's for the person to vividly recall childhood events from fifty years previous, but not be able to recall meeting someone two hours ago. We now know that Alzheimer's patients have a "short-circuiting" of brain cells in the hippocampus area of the brain, the area where short-term memory and learning take place. These effects appear to result from brain cell damage associated with elevated levels of "heavy metals" like aluminum, and the formation of "plaques" composed of a protein called beta-amyloid. Subsequently, cells start getting "tangled up" inside with "filbrils" of a protein called tau, resulting in what are called "neurofibrillary tangles." Interestingly, aluminum causes the accumulation of tau protein and beta-amyloid protein in experimental animals, and induces brain cell death (apoptosis) in vivo as well as in vitro, but is not the major causative factor. [8]

There also appears to be failure of the mitochondrial energy factories within the cells, so there is insufficient energy for the cell to do its work and stay alive. No drugs are currently available to either prevent or correct these biochemical defects. Present drugs, though widely advertised and prescribed, provide only mild temporary "improvement," and theoretically could even be accelerating cell death. Since the brain cells can utilize either glucose or ketones to produce needed cell energy (ATP), early Alzheimer's can be successfully treated with medium chain triglycerides (MCT oil). (Find MCT oil at www.pipingrock.com)

We're now ready to review some of the exciting studies done on Bacopa.

- A 2002 Australian double-blind study of memory functions in 76 adults did not change previous (long-term) memories, but significantly enhanced memory of new information. (20)

- One of Bacopa's active nutrients (Bacoside A) was found to enhance the brain's antioxidant defenses, increasing superoxide dismutase (SOD), catalase, and glutathione peroxidase – protecting brain cell (mitochondrial) energy production. (21)

- Bacopa extract was found to increase superoxide dismutase (SOD), catalase, and glutathione peroxidase activities in all brain regions tested, including hippocampus (the principal learning and memory center), being superior to an "anti-aging" drug (deprenyl) that increased brain antioxidants, but not in the all-important hippocampus. (22)

- A 2001 Australian double-blind study in healthy human subjects showed that Bacopa "significantly improved....learning rate and memory consolidation."(23)

- A 2003 Italian study showed Bacopa to be a strong antioxidant which could prevent DNA damage. The authors felt this "may explain the reported anti-stress, immune supporting, cognition-facilitating, anti-inflammatory and anti-aging effects produced by Bacopa in experimental animals and in clinical situations ..." [24]

- A 2008 study from India showed Bacopa to have more effective anti-inflammation activity than non-steroidal anti-inflammatory drugs like Indocin. It inhibited COX-2 and LOX (lipoxygenase), and down-regulated TNF-alpha (inflammation inducers). [25]

- A 2008 Australian double-blind study in 62 normal adults showed significantly improved memory performance and spatial working memory accuracy. [26]

- A 2008 Portland, Oregon randomized double-blind study testing Bacopa in 48 aged adults (average 73.5 years) showed broad improvement in "cognitive performance, anxiety, and depression." [27]

Turning to Alzheimer's specifically, and the known brain-toxic effects of Aluminum in brain tissue, two recent studies with Bacopa are of interest.

- A 2006 New Delhi study using aluminum chloride to generate neurotoxicity in rat brain hippocampus showed that co-administration of Bacopa extract prevented intraneuronal lipofuscin accumulation and brain cell death in this critical learning and memory region. (28) (Note: lipofucsin is the "age pigment" that causes the brown "liver spots" seen on skin of aged people, but which also occur in the aging brain.)

- A 2008 university study, in vitro, showed that Bacopa protected cortical brain cells from beta-amyloid-induced cell death. (29)

On a different note, a 2001 study demonstrated Bacopa to have a "stabilizing" effect on mast cells. Mast cells are the principle source of histamine release when destabilized (activated by allergens). (30) Thus, Bacopa may play a role in controlling allergic reactions like asthma, or autoimmune disorders like arthritis.

And so, is Bacopa nature's best protector of the brain, a great memory enhancer, the answer for ADHD and Alzheimer's, an effective antihistamine, an immune system rebalancer, an answer for autoimmune disorders – or all the above? The answers are not yet final. But that Bacopa is a fine addition to neutraceutical formulations there seems little doubt.

But let's move on to another exciting power nutrient – Astaxanthin.

Nine

Power Nutrient – Astaxanthin

Astaxanthin is the bright red color seen in red sockeye salmon, in boiled lobster, and in shrimp. It is a red pigment, in the same carotenoid category as the orange pigment beta carotene, which gives carrots their color.

Carotenoids are antioxidant free-radical scavengers with many health benefits. But Astaxanthin is unique among the 700 members of the carotenoid class of antioxidants. It is harvested in pristine Hawaiian waters from the micro algae Hematococcus pluvialis. Eating algae is how salmon, shrimp, and lobster get their supply of this important antioxidant. Four ounces of sockeye salmon contains about 4 mg of Astaxanthin and is the currently recommended daily intake for this nutrient. (31, 32)

So why have we included Astaxanthin in our list? A simple answer is that it is an all natural, non-toxic, super antioxidant with impressive science supporting it. Let's review a few of the relevant in vivo and in vitro studies:

- A 2005 study from the International Research Center in Japan showed that Astaxanthin "can exert beneficial effects in protection against hypertension and stroke and in improving memory in vascular dementia." (33)

- A 2006 Harvard study found that the cardio-toxicity of the popular anti-inflammatory drug Vioxx was caused by oxidation of LDL cholesterol and oxidation of heart cells. But this oxidation damage (free-radical damage) "can be blocked by the potent antioxidant Astaxanthin." (34)

- A 2004 Washington State University review of carotenoid action on the in vivo immune response (with reference to lutein, lycopene, and Astaxanthin) revealed that these substances enhance both cell-mediated and humoral immune responses in animals and humans. As such they play important roles in control of "diseases such as cancer, cardiovascular and neurodegenerative diseases and aging." A double-blind study by these authors showed Astaxanthin to both enhance immune function and decrease DNA damage from free-radicals. [35]

• A 1994 Japanese study showed the superiority of Astaxanthin to other carotenoids in prevention of transitional-cell carcinoma (bladder cancer) in mice. [36] Other authors have shown Astaxanthin to also have preventive effects on breast cancer and colon cancer. [37]

What we can conclude is that Astaxanthin is a carotenoid super antioxidant, a natural substance from clean ocean waters and may play an important role in keeping us healthy.

Let's move on now to a very exciting power nutrient that has been making news in major research centers from Harvard to the National Institute on Aging.

Ten

Power Nutrient – Resveratrol

One of the most exciting areas of current neutraceutical research involves the polyphenol Resveratrol. Why is this area of research so hot? Because resveratrol is starting to look like a true "fountain of youth," a real longevity substance. Resveratrol is found naturally in red wines and probably partly explains the known health benefits attributed to red wine.

The current burst of interest started with the 1990's research from Dr. David Sinclair's lab at Harvard. He found he could duplicate the known life-lengthening benefits of a calorie-restricted diet, by giving resveratrol to overfed rats that usually die young with arthritis, cardiovascular disease, and senile dementia. Dr. Sinclair's work has shown that resveratrol's benefits

may be less associated with its antioxidant properties, than with its abilities as a communication molecule acting upon a cells genetic activity. By 2004,
his research was showing resveratrol to have a regu-
latory effect on the SIRT-1 gene – a disease and age
regulating gene. All the facts are not yet in on how
SIRT-1 and other associated genes like Fox03 and p53
produce their wellness and anti-aging effects. But one
thing seems clear – resveratrol plays a major role in
these effects. Resveratrol-mediated Sirtuin activation
is now believed responsible for some level of protection against age-associated disorders like atherosclerosis (heart disease and stroke), metabolic syndrome
and diabetes, cancer, and neurodegenerative processes
(Parkinson's, Alzheimer's).

So explosive and exciting is the current worldwide
research on resveratrol that we will here review just a
sampling of recent scientific studies:

- In a 2008 review article entitled "Trans-
  resveratrol: a magic elixir of eternal youth?"
  from University of Santiago, Spain, the author
  explores some of the mechanisms by which
  trans-resveratrol may act as an anti-aging
  agent. He also summarizes the in vitro and
  in vivo studies showing trans-resveratrol's

anti-inflammatory, antioxidant, platelet antiaggregatory and anticarcinogenic properties. (38)

- An important 2008 research study from University of Nottingham, UK demonstrated that resveratrol "has potent effects at a physiological concentration (0.1 microm) that would be expected to result in vasodilation and therefore help reduce blood pressure and the risk of cardiovascular diseases." (39) (Early studies had used much larger amounts of resveratrol than occur physiologically from red wine drinking. But in animal studies, modest increases of Sirtuin 1 protein improved cardiac health, while greater than a 7.5 fold increase in Sirtuin 1 gene protein <u>induced</u> heart failure in laboratory mice! [Circulation Research 100; 1512-21,2007]). This U.K. study showed resveratrol up-regulated 233 genes, and down regulated the expression of 363 genes, all at these very small physiologic levels, demonstrating again that foods we eat have important DNA genetic modifying activities!

- The above noted U.K. study also showed that resveratrol (0.1 microm) "significantly increased the expression of the gene encoding endothelial Nitric Oxide synthase (eNOS), which synthesizes the vasodilator molecule Nitric Oxide (NO), and decreases the expression of the potent vasoconstrictor, endothelin-1 (ET-1)." (39) (An interesting "foot note" here is that Dr. Louis Ignarro won the Nobel Prize in Medicine in 1998 for his discovery of Nitric Oxide and its vital role in preserving arterial health. Based on NO activity, he wrote a 2005 book entitled "NO More Heart Disease" wherein he believes that the heart disease that kills 50% of Americans could be prevented by substances that increase Nitric Oxide (NO) production in the cells that line the interior of our blood vessels! Which, within the blood vessels, is precisely what resveratrol does!

- An interesting 2006 in vitro study from University of Coimbra, Portugal, demonstrated that resveratrol increased intracellular glutathione content of bovine arterial endothelial cells, thus preventing peroxynitrite free-radical damage to arteries, one of the causes of atherosclerosis and heart disease. (40) (Glutathione is the body's most important cell-preserving antioxidant, found in all human cells)

- A 2009 research review from University of Barcelona entitled: "Resveratrol and neurode-generative diseases" considers resveratrol an ideal neuroprotective substance to both prevent and possibly treat neurological disorders like Parkinson's disease and Alzheimer's disease. (41)

- An important 2009 in-vivo study from the Department of Neurosciences, Cornell University utilizing Alzheimer's mice showed a 90% reduction of beta-amyloid plaque formation in the hippocampus area of the brain after 45 days feeding "clinically feasible dosages of resveratrol!" (42) This is the brain area most important for memory and learning, the area most-damaged by plaque in Alzheimer's disease. This study, interestingly, showed no activation of SIRT-1, supporting a view that resveratrol may act in multiple ways beyond Sirtuin activities.

- Important research from the Cleveland Clinic published in 2009 elucidates the "trapping" process by which "foam" cells (macrophage white blood cells filled with oxidized LDL cholesterol particles) create the atherosclerotic plaque causing heart attacks and strokes.

Resveratrol can not only block the formation of foam-cell plaque, but can facilitate the release of these foam cells from arterial walls, reversing the process. (43)

• Referencing the above Cleveland Clinic research, Linda Curtiss, PhD, an immunologist from Scripps Research Institute (La Jolla, CA) in an editorial published in March 12, 2009 issue of the New England Journal of Medicine, states:

> "Atherosclerosis is reversible and involves the removal of trapped cholesterol-loaded foam-cell macrophages from the arterial intima. A recent study by Park and Colleagues showed that these foam cells are trapped by interaction with oxidized low-density lipoprotein (LDL) and can be remobilized by dynamic exposure to key antioxidants such as resveratrol..." (44)

Thus resveratrol shows a variety of important health-enhancing activities including blocking oxidation of LDL cholesterol (the necessary initial step to produce atherosclerotic plaque), enhancing glutathione production, protecting brain and nervous system from degenerative diseases, helping reverse insulin resistance (insulin resistance is the initial step to developing diabetes), acting to reverse atherosclerosis, enhancing intravascular nitric oxide production to lower high blood pressure, and activating the SIRT-1 longevity gene. While research in the next few years will modify some of our present knowledge, there is little question that resveratrol is a disease-fighting, anti-aging superstar.

Eleven

Power Nutrient –
Grape Seed Extract

N ow, you might ask, what good could possibly come from those little hard gray seeds we think are such an annoyance when eating grapes – at least before some clever scientist found a way to genetically modify grapes so they would grow without seeds. (But recall that from that little seed a new vine can grown, and without seeds the fruit cannot reproduce!)

So what's in the little seed that makes it so nutritionally interesting? Well, get ready for one of the most colorful journeys into recent scientific discovery.

The story starts in the winter of 1536, when the French explorer Jacques Cartier and his crew were exploring the St. Lawrence River in Canada. The river froze, trapping his ship and crew. Living on salted meat, but lacking fresh fruits or vegetables, they fell victim to the deadly scourge of scurvy, a vitamin C deficiency disease. Twenty-five of his crew died before friendly Quebec Indians shared with them a tea brewed from pine tree bark indigenous to that area ("Maritime Pine Bark"). Miraculously, this stopped the scurvy, and Cartier recorded this remarkable event in his ship's log. No one had any idea what it could be in pine tree bark to so amazingly cure a deadly disease like scurvy.

The story now moves ahead 400 years, when a French scientist named Jacques Masquelier happened to read Jacques Cartier's log book, and wondered what might be in pine bark to produce these remarkable cures. He went to work and discovered substances in pine bark called proanthocyanidins. He also found that there were various types of proanthocyanidin molecules and that the smaller ("oligo" from the Greek, meaning "little") molecules were far more potent "healers" than the larger forms. And so were born the Oligomeric Proanthocyanidins, otherwise known simply as OPCs.

Dr. Masquelier found in lab animals that these OPC's caused their blood vessels to double in strength! Within just a couple hours following oral intake!

Continuing his OPC studies, Dr. Masquelier found to his surprise that grape seeds – tons of which were regularly thrown away after pressing the juice from grapes for wine making –were an even richer source of these OPC's! So he now had a cheap, common source, and no longer had to strip the bark from pine trees! With his lab in Bordeaux where the great Grand Cru Cabernet wines are produced, he had an abundance of grape seeds. Not surprisingly, he patented his process for OPC extraction from both pine bark and from grape seeds – the grape seed process in 1970. While these original patented extracts have remained quite expensive, other companies now produce grape seed extract by slightly modified methods, and thus at much lower cost to consumers.

So this brings us to the question of what's so re-markable about grape seed extract OPCs, what do they do, how do they work, what's the current science of their in vivo and in vitro effects.

Grape seed extracts high in OPCs offer some of nature's most powerful wellness and healing benefits. Consider the following:

- A 2009 University of California, Davis placebo-controlled double-blind study in human adults with the metabolic syndrome showed that treatment with grape seed extract would lower both systolic and diastolic blood pressure. (45)

Let me stop here and explain what "metabolic syndrome" is all about. So-called **Metabolic Syndrome** (also known as Syndrome X) is a relatively recent "disease" label given to those people – male and female – who show 3 of the following:

1. a fat abdomen

2. elevated serum triglycerides

3. low serum HDLs (the "good" cholesterol)

4. high blood pressure

5. elevated serum glucose (FBS-fasting blood sugar)

What's so important about this condition is that most overweight people already have – or will have – metabolic syndrome. And metabolic syndrome is a precursor to diabetes, heart attacks, strokes, cancers, Alzheimer's and arthritis! Since 70% of American adults and 30% of children are overweight, this clearly is the major health problem in the United States, and in many other countries. *Simply put, Metabolic Syndrome is a serious metabolic derangement that provides the platform for almost all our chronic degenerative and life-shortening diseases.* And the cause of Metabolic Syndrome is also now clear: America's addiction to white sugar, white flour, white rice, and white potato – the soda pop, sports drinks, donuts, pies, boxed breakfast cereals, pancakes, cookies, crackers, muffins, candy bars, ice cream, French fries, hash-browns, potato chips – and hundreds other destructive "foods" that line the shelves of supermarkets everywhere.

But back to grape seed extract. The fact that grape seed extract lowers blood pressure in Metabolic Syndrome implies that grape seed extract plays an important role in trying to bring balance and health back toward normal. We might ask, how does grape seed extract lower blood pressure? The answer is a rather interesting one.

The 1998 Nobel Prize in Medicine was won by three American pharmacologists, Dr. Robert F. Furchgott of New York, Dr. Louis Ignarro of Los Angeles, and Dr. Ferid Murad of Houston. Their discovery was for nitric oxide, a gas which acts as a critical "signaling molecule" within the cardiovascular system, within the immune system and within the nervous system. Lining all the arteries and veins of the cardiovascular system, for example, is a thin single layer of cells called endothelium cells. It is these endothelium cells that each can produce this gas, nitric oxide.

Dr. Furghott had first published a paper in 1980 describing some mysterious substance which caused blood vessels to relax (vasodilate). (46) As arteries dilate to a larger size, this causes blood pressure to drop. Conversely, anything that causes arteries to constrict will raise the blood pressure. Furchgott called this mysterious vasodilator substance "endothelium–derived relaxing factor" or EDRF.

And it wasn't until 1986 that Drs. Furchgott, Ignarro, and Salvador Moncada independently showed the mystery substance EDRF to be nitric oxide gas. This small gaseous molecule causes blood vessel smooth muscle to relax – resulting in dilation of the vessel and lowering of blood pressure.

And getting back to grape seed extract, it is the oligomeric proanthocyanidins that in fact stimulate nitric oxide production and play several very important roles to keep the cardiovascular system healthy. (47)

Two factoids here are of interest:

1. The brain is one of the richest sources of nitric oxide activity, and nitric oxide may play a major role in maintaining memory and keeping the brain healthy.

2. Nitric oxide is what makes the firefly glow!

And that's only the beginning of the science behind grape seed OPCs.

- A 2005 in vivo study from Terragona, Spain showed that grape seed proanthocyanidins

(OPCs) lowered serum triglyceride levels, LDL ("bad") cholesterol levels, and Apolipoprotein B levels, thus decreasing the likelihood of athero-sclerosis, heart attacks, and strokes. [48] Elevated triglycerides, LDL, and Apolipoprotein B are all considered important indicators of increased heart attack risk. Especially significant here is the lowering of the Apolipoprotein B level. Elevated Apolipoprotien B levels are now considered a far more reliable indicator of heart at-tack risk than are LDL ("bad") cholesterol and total cholesterol values!

- A well done 2003 study from Creighton University (Omaha) – done on animals and hu-mans – outlined several molecular pathways by which grape seed extract provides protec-tion from atherosclerosis and heart attacks. [49] Grape seed provided far better antioxidant protection than did Vitamin C, Vitamin E, or beta-carotene. And it significantly reduced oxidized LDL (oxidized LDL is considered the initial "bad stuff" that starts the formation of dangerous plaque in the arteries – plaque that leads to heart attacks and strokes). They concluded that grape seed extract could play an important role to keep arteries and heart healthy.

- A 2008 in vivo study from Spain further elucidated the complex cellular mechanisms by which grape seed OPCs control cholesterol metabolism, protect the cardiovascular system, and are able to down regulate (turn off) several genes that create "bad" cholesterol. (50) What's important here is that grape seed nutrients were clearly shown to regulate one's DNA – the genes that regulate all cellular and organ function. In other words, grape seed extract was able – in very positive, health promoting ways – to influence the essence of life itself. Not the way toxic synthetic drugs like statins (Lipitor, Crestor, and a dozen others) interfere with normal liver and muscle function, but by regulating the genes that control healthy cholesterol metabolism, to keep it healthy without toxic damage. This is no small issue, when one considers that statin drugs are the largest selling drugs in the world – to lower cholesterol, when total cholesterol level is not really the problem! It's oxidized LDL that's the major issue. And preventing oxidation of LDL is what antioxidants do, not statin drugs! "Poisoning" the liver to block the production of cholesterol is a bizarre misdirection of efforts, based on a fifty-year old mistaken belief that cholesterol is what causes plaques and atherosclerosis.

But lets continue our exploration of benefits from grape seed extract.

Let's shift gears from cardiovascular health to brain health. We know that heart attacks are the leading cause of death, but Alzheimer's dementia is probably what aging people fear the most. Interestingly, there is no present drug that can prevent or effectively treat Alzheimer's disease! Alzheimer's disease is characterized by progressive neuro-degeneration with loss of cognitive and memory functions.

More interestingly, recent studies with grape seed extract show some exciting results not only to prevent Alzheimer's but also to treat it.

- A 2008 in vivo study from Mount Sinai School of Medicine (New York) showed that in Alzheimer mice suffering dementia and memory deficits, grape seed extract will "significantly inhibit amyloid beta-protein aggregation (in vitro), and significantly (stop) cognitive deterioration...in the brain." (in vivo). (51)

Let's explain here what we know about Alzheimer's at this point in time. About 50 years of Alzheimer's research has shown that there are probably five major abnormalities currently believed to play roles in development of Alzheimer's dementia:

1. Deposition of "neurofibrillary tangles" in brain neurons. Neurons like all cells have a microtubular protein skeleton. When the microtubular protein called "tau" is not formed properly, it results in twisted filaments called neurofibrillary tangles, which play a role in malfunction and death of brain cells in Alzheimer's disease.

2. "Beta-amyloid plaques" are another constant finding in Alzheimer's disease brains. Current science believes that this amyloid deposition to form a large brain plaque, is an "assembly process" of smaller amyloid fragments.

3. Atherosclerosis of cerebral blood vessels, impairing normal blood flow and oxygenation of brain cells.

4. Impaired brain energy production involving the mitochondria (small "energy factories") within brain cells. Damage to mitochondria produces "abnormal mitochondrial dynamics."

5. Oxidation (free-radical damage) and inflammation, which damage cell and mitochondrial membranes and DNA.

As if these confirmed causes weren't enough, heavy metal toxicity (Aluminum, Mercury, Lead, Iron), pesticide-fungicide toxicities, and VOCs (volatile organic compounds from paints, solvents, synthetic carpeting, etc) may also be implicated.

Most likely there are a dozen or so "causes" and processes involved over a lifetime that create the neuro degeneration seen in this disease. This is one reason why the idea of a single-chemical synthetic drug that will prevent or cure Alzheimer's is terribly unrealistic.

All of which gets us back to our review of grape seed extract benefits. Is it possible that the hundreds of "nutrients" in grape seed extract can play a role in keeping the brain healthy?

- A 2008 study from the Mount Sinai School of Medicine (New York), using a specially-developed mouse model of Alzheimer's Disease (AD) showed that grape seed extract "significantly attenuates AD-type cognitive deterioration coincidentally with reduced (amyloid deposition) in the brain."[52] The eight scientists involved in this important study conclude: "Our study suggests that grape seed derived polyphenolics may be useful agents to prevent or treat AD."

- A later 2008 in vitro study from UCLA School of Medicine, using sophisticated intracellular imaging techniques including electron microscopy, determined that grape seed extract inhibited the assembly of beta amyloid plaque and protected cells from its toxic effects. These authors conclude: "These data suggest that (grape seed extract) is worthy of consideration as a therapeutic agent for AD." (53)

Finally, we will turn to grape seed extract as a useful agent to keep the intestinal tract healthy, and a possible role in thereby preventing colon cancer, one of our deadliest common cancers. In fact, colorectal cancer is the third most common cancer in both men and women.

- A 2008 in vitro study from University of Colorado used three different cultured human colorectal cancer cell lines, and tested whether grape seed extract could affect these cancers. Surprisingly, in all three types, cancer growth was "strongly" inhibited, and there was an increase in death of cancer cells. (54)

While in vitro studies do not automatically translate to clinical efficacy, they do represent an important early indicator of possible success in human clinical trails.

In summary, we note that grape seed extract contains hundreds of plant nutrients vitally important to good health, and may provide protection from some of our most serious human diseases.

Grape seed extracts can vary in quality and efficacy. My recommendation: Meganatural-BP or similar product.

Twelve

Power Nutrient – Curcumin

This, the eighth of our list of power nutrients, is a rising star in the world of health-giving botanicals. Curcumin – and its contained curcuminoids – is found in turmeric root, a spice used in Indian curries. Curcumin has an intense yellow-orange color, is used as a coloring agent in many foods, and has long been part of traditional Indian Ayurvedic Medicine.

Curcumin has been shown to have antioxidant, anti-inflammation, antiviral, antibacterial, antifungal and anticancer activities.

- A 2007 review of curcumin's many benefits from M.D. Anderson Cancer Center (Houston) points out that curcumin has "natural" actions that at least 8 current synthetic drugs try to emulate. The authors conclude that "considering the recent scientific bandwagon that multi-targeted therapy is better than mono-targeted therapy for most diseases, curcumin can be considered an ideal 'Spice for Life'." (55)

- In other words, curcumin has been found to act beneficially in a wide range of body systems and metabolic processes, explaining why Ayurvedic Medicine for centuries has used turmeric root (curcumin) to effectively treat a wide range of human illnesses.

- An important 2005 in vivo study from UCLA School of Medicine, used aged Alzheimer's disease mice with advanced amyloid accumulation in the brain and found that curcumin would block fibril and plaque formation, and could <u>reduce</u> amyloid already present. This remarkable reversal of Alzheimer's led the researchers to conclude: "These data suggest that low dose curcumin effectively disaggregates (i.e. dissolves) beta amyloid, as well as prevents fibril and (plaque) formation, supporting the rationale for curcumin use in clinical trials preventing or treating Alzheimer's Disease." (56)

On another note, recent research is implicating iron accumulation in the body as perhaps a major cause of many diseases, free radical formation, and shortened lifespan.

⇒ A 2008 report from Wake Forest School of Medicine (Winston-Salem, NC) points out that: "Curcumin is not only a free radical scavenger, but also binds metals, particularly iron and copper, and can function as an iron chelator." (57)

So, while numerous human trials get under way, extensive research strongly supports curcumin as a many faceted, and impressive health-promoting botanical. My recommendation, look for the BCM-95 form of curcumin such as Super Bio Curcumin from Life Extension (www.lifeextension.com)

Thirteen

Power Nutrients – Adaptogens

One of the truly great scientific accomplishments of the 20th century was the discovery by Soviet scientists of "super herbs" called Adaptogens. Adaptogen research began in the late 1940s, and by the 1970s their use became a force in the USSR.

Unheralded here in the U.S. because of our commitment to pharmaceutical drugs, it was Adaptogens that propelled the USSR to dominance of Olympic Gold, to world chess championships, and allowed them to send a cosmonaut into high-stress space travel a full year ahead of the U.S.'s John Glen.

Twenty years, 1200 of their best scientists, and massive human trials testing whole factories of workers or even entire city populations – allowed them to locate and test thousands of herbal plants to discover those few that had powerful attributes to protect humans from the damaging effects of STRESS. They named these non-toxic, super plant extracts "Adaptogens" because they allowed recipients to adjust and adapt to high stress effects on human physiology – all without the toxic "side effects " so common to pharmaceuticals.

Soviet scientists had been impressed with the stress discoveries of Hungarian-Canadian scientist, Dr. Hans Selye, who first showed in the 1940s that stressful events could produce significant and damaging effects to the brain, muscles, and cardiovascular systems of animals and humans.

Dr. Israel I. Brekhman headed the soviet studies, all done in secret and not published in standard scientific journals.

I first learned about Adaptogens as a Vice President of the company that first brought these remarkable herbs to the United States in the early 1990s. Another Vice President hired by the company had been the Head of Research and Training for the Soviet track and field Olympic teams, Dr. B. Tabachnik. It was from Dr. Tabachnik that I would learn the inside story of Adaptogens, and their amazing attributes. He shared with me original research papers done by Dr Brekhman and other top Soviet scientists, work he and I would share with audiences across the U.S., as we represented the company and its products.

Rather than single synthetic chemicals that characterize all pharmaceutical drugs, Adaptogens were found to each posses hundreds of natural plant "phytochemicals" that worked in harmony to rebalance metabolism and protect the body from stress damage. Brekhman was acclaimed a Soviet national hero, though his work remained little known in the West until the 1990's when the Soviet system collapsed.

So what are some of these few super-plants and what do they do for us?

The primary Adaptogens from Soviet science included Eleutherococus, Rhodiola, Schizandra, Aralia, Rhaponticum and a few others.

Indian Ayurvedic medicine has also made Adaptogen claims for Ashwaghanda.

Long-term chronic stress, we now know, produces muscle wasting, accumulation of belly fat, memory loss, brain damage, immune system suppression, adrenal gland burnout, and premature aging.

Adaptogens address ALL these issues.

While most of the original Soviet research is still difficult to access on Western research databases, I will share one documented study that so impressed me.

It was a seven-year study done on hundreds of high-stress heavy equipment drivers, (1973-1979) and measured the annual incidence of influenza, hypertension, and coronary heart disease attacks, resulting in days loss of work.[59] The men were required to take just 2 cc of the herbal extract (Eleuthero) daily. At the beginning of the study there was a 55% annual illness rate, resulting in days of lost work. By the third year this rate of illness had dropped to 37%, rather impressive. But by the fifth year, the illness rate had dropped to 15%, and when the study concluded in the seventh year, the annual illness rate had dropped to 3% ! This remarkable result suggested strongly that the longer a person remained on this Adaptogen, the better someone's heath became! No drug, diet, discipline, or vitamin-mineral supplement has been shown to achieve such a result!

These super-herbs are the "base substances" upon which a healthy diet and other supplements best work. They are my #1 secret to great health and long life. Why? Because they deal with the #1 cause of aging: Stress damage, in ways no other nutritional supplement will. Adaptogens are simply the most powerful Health Restorers on earth!

While several Adaptogen-containing supplements have appeared in the marketplace, I believe only those closest to the Russian original formulations, are recommended.

The one I take daily is "LHL Formula #1" and can be ordered on the internet at: www.LHLcode.com

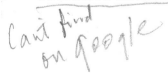

Can't find on google

Fourteen

Putting It All Together

We've discussed nine power nutrients, carefully selected to protect human cells and organs from the influences that are now believed to underlie all the chronic degenerative diseases of aging, and of the aging process itself.

These aging influences have recently been shown to include oxidation, inflammation, dysregulation of mitochondrial energy production, and unbalanced neuro-endocrine signaling. In other words, the millions of biochemical reactions taking place every second in our bodies start to short-circuit, accumulate toxins, attack our genetic DNA and result in illness, fatigue, and degenerative diseases.

The body's way of protecting us from these destructive processes is to use food nutrients to provide energy, balance, and detoxification. To maintain this great balanced symphony of life requires quality foods and supplements, modest exercise, regular sleep, stress reduction, and avoiding toxins.

Modern nutritional science is showing that carefully selected dietary supplements can play a major role in preserving and restoring optimal vitality and wellness. This is "preventive medicine" at its best. True preventive medicine requires lifestyle choices that maintain cells, organs, and systems in youthful patterns of function. This includes the cardiovascular system, the brain and nervous system, the hormone-endocrine system, the immune system, and the spiritual-emotional-attitudinal system. Modern medical care does its best to manage serious disease after it occurs, and uses pharmaceuticals to bring relief of symptoms. Nutrition-based "preventive medicine" seeks to prevent the disease by correcting the cause.

These nine natural factors are a carefully-selected group of power nutrients shown to positively influence biochemical processes in ways to maintain optimal health and to move abnormal functions back toward normal. One foundational way this happens is via the thin, single layer of cells lining the body's 100,000 miles of blood vessels. (58) These "endothelium" cells are the dynamic surface through which all nutrients pass to the cells of all organs – whether brain, heart, liver, or muscles. Nobel Prize Winner, Sir John Vane, called the endothelium the "maestro of circulation."

Keeping endothelium cells healthy is a key to wellness, one that several of these power ingredients address.

Adding Berries To The Diet: Dark-colored berries have high anthocyanin and polyphenol levels. They reduce inflammation and oxidation, support balanced immune function, and are natural COX-2 inhibitors of inflammation. They each contain more than a hundred phytonutrients to support energy production and protect cardiovascular health. Ditto for northern arctic berries.

Glutathione Generators: Glutathione is the body's master wellness molecule. Its many functions include:

⇒ Antioxidant, and anti-inflammatory

⇒ Regenerates other antioxidants like vitamin C, vitamin E, vitamin A, and alpha lipoic acid

⇒ Is a major liver detoxifier

⇒ Chelates heavy metals like mercury, lead, aluminum, cadmium, arsenic, and iron

⇒ Prevents formation of skin-aging substances called Advanced Glycation End Products (AGES).

Interestingly, in all human diseases, body levels of glutathione are found to be low. But glutathione is not as bioavailable when taken orally. To improve intracellular glutathione levels requires taking glutathione *precursors* by mouth. These include nutrients like N-Acetyl Cysteine, and alpha lipoic acid.

Bacopa Monnieri: One of the most revered herbs of ancient Ayervedic medicine - a true brain tonic. Human clinical studies have now shown that Bacopa significantly improves learning and memory, increases brain cell antioxidants, lessens anxiety and depression. Good studies from Australia, India, and the U.S. have all shown Bacopa to be an effective non-toxic memory improver!

Astaxanthin: A super carotenoid antioxidant derived from Hawaiian algae. It is the red color in sockeye salmon and in boiled lobster. Its oxygen-radical neutralizing power is 500 times greater than that of alpha tocopherol (vitamin E). Epidemiological studies show a correlation between carotenoid intake and a reduced incidence of coronary heart disease and certain cancers – and increased resistance to viral, bacterial, fungal, and parasitic infections. Astaxanthin provides strong support to the immune system.

Curcumin: Derived from turmeric root and used extensively in Indian curries, this plant substance is a rising star in the world of botanical nutrients. While definitive human studies are still being undertaken, research to date shows it to be a powerful antioxidant, anti-inflammatory, and genetic modifier that may play important roles to combat cardiovascular disease, cancer, senile dementias and auto-inflammatory diseases.

Resveratrol: The recently discovered anti-aging superstar. Resveratrol is a polyphenol found in the skins of grapes and red wines. It is a broad-spectrum antioxidant which increases the body's own major antioxidants (SOD, catalase, glutathione reductase, vitamin C, vitamin E, and others), and prevents damage to genetic DNA. It helps keep endothelium cells healthy, activates the SIRT-1 longevity gene, and may act to reverse atherosclerosis.

Grape Seed Extract: Is a rich source of oligomeric proanthocyanidins (OPCs). Studies show it can reduce likelihood of senile dementias and Alzheimer's disease. It also supports cardiovascular health, helps lower high blood pressure, and induces the important "signaling molecule" nitric oxide within the arteries to keep arteries flexible and healthy. GSE can lower LDL (bad cholesterol) levels and reduce serum triglyceride levels, thus reducing likelihood of heart attack and stroke.

Green Tea and Green Tree Extract: A potent antioxidant 200 times stronger than vitamin E. It has anti-viral properties and blocks carcinogens and cancer metastases. It reduces the risk of bladder, pancreatic, ovarian, and prostate cancers. It protects brain health and reduces the risk of Parkinson's disease. Because it's a thermogenic, it can also be a mild aid for weight loss.

Adaptogens: A collection of thoroughly-tested super herbs discovered by top Soviet scientists starting in the late 1940s. These safe, and non-toxic extracts were shown they:

⇒ Block the damaging effects of stress on human physiology.

⇒ Improved brain function and memory

⇒ Strengthened immune function to protect against colds, flus, and other diseases

⇒ Improved physical performance for athletes

⇒ Helped re-balance all body systems to move abnormal function back to normal

⇒ Kept improving health the longer they were used

Fifteen

Your Spiritual –
Emotional Health

"And with long life will I satisfy them."

- Psalm 91:16

We all know that our emotions and attitudes impact our health, and determine much of our happiness in life.

But did you know that your emotions and attitudes:

- Strengthen or weaken your immune system and thus influence how many colds, flus, and other diseases you will get?

- Influence how much inflammation you have in your body, inflammation that leads to a large variety of diseases?

- Influence the length of your telomeres – the small caps on the ends of your chromosomes, caps that can lengthen or shorten from effects of emotions, caps that protect chromosomal DNA from damage and mutations to cancer, caps that determine how long your cells will live?

- Can turn on or turn off health-enhancing genes, or health-damaging genes?

- Can even influence intestinal health and the ratio of good to bad bacteria that inhabit your gut?

Hard to believe, but true, and with good science to support it!

And "emotional" health also has important "spiritual" connections. In other words, the quality of your spiritual belief also impacts human health. Many are familiar with the Bible, Old Testament verse (Isaiah 40:31):

"But those who wait upon the Lord shall renew their strength; they shall mount up with wings like eagles, they shall run and not be weary, they shall walk and not faint."

And from Psalm 91:1 "Those who dwell in the shelter of the Most High will experience calmness of spirit in the shadow of the Almighty."

Or the oft-quoted words of Jesus (John 10:10):

"I have come that you might have life, and have it more abundantly."

And again (John 8:12)

"I am the light of the world. Whoever follows me will never walk in darkness, but will have the light of life."

On a more secular level, few books on health and "self-healing" have equaled the 1979 classic by Saturday Review Editor-in-Chief, Norman Cousins, entitled "Anatomy of an Illness" and subtitled, "Reflections on Healing and Regeneration." Cousins' pain and severe arthritic inflammation were brought under control, he believes by "use of laughter" and "cultivation of the will to live" by both himself and by his physician. This is a powerful, and beautifully written, testimony to the importance of mind, emotions, and beliefs.

Few doubt that "as a man thinks, so is he." In other words, thoughts that go through our heads most persistently will create the world in which we live !

Being filled with anger, frustration, hatred and the need to dominate others will all produce a very different person – and level of physical health – than one ennobled with joy, smiles, happiness, compassion, and an ability to "put the best construction on everything."

We're not talking here about unrealistic blind optimism in the face of black disaster. We are talking about a positive mindset that as an old Chinese proverb opines, "Tis better to light one small candle, than to curse the darkness."

In this modern age of instant international communication, no one doubts the high level of darkness, destruction, and evil forces that dominate so much of our world. And while putting ones head in the sand of denial is foolish and irresponsible, we nonetheless can remain sober and favor an upbeat kindness, love, and generosity of spirit to brighten both ours and others lives.

Remember, "kindness can't be given away, it just keeps coming back."

Thomas Merton, an American Trappist Monk, in his spiritual masterpiece, "No Man is an Island," says it so well in the title of Chapter One, "Love can be kept only by being given away."

The rush and incessant activity of modern life often undoes the quietness and calmness of mind needed for purposeful pursuits that support health and healing. Grabbing a cola drink, a bag of chips, and a donut "on the run " will sabotage health and happiness. They're no substitute for taking the time to enjoy a salad, an organic apple or orange, and a cup of plain low-fat yogurt!

Maharishi Mahesh Yogi's Transcendental Mediation technique allows the mind to rest and find an inner core of peace that slows today's madness and mayhem. And studies have shown that Transcendental Meditation, twenty minutes once or twice a day, brings substantial health benefits. A study published in the journal Circulation found that Transcendental Meditation can lower blood pressure, reduce the risk of heart attack or stroke, and reduce the risk for Alzheimer's Disease by improving brain-cell activity. This form of meditation creates a state of profound rest and relaxation, and calms the mind to achieve a state of inner peace, without needing to use concentration or effort.

Combining healthy emotions with positive spiritual experiences and mind-quieting meditation-relaxation are all an important part of your Living Healthier Longer program.

Sixteen

The Living Healthier
Longer Program

By now I hope it's clear that you must take control of your own health. Below is the final distillation of concepts and dosages for those ideas and power nutrients we've discussed.

In its simplest terms, virtually all the chronic degenerative diseases of aging are the result of:

1. **High-sugar, high-carbohydrate diets**.

2. **Toxins** from cigarette smoking, the thousands of pesticides, preservatives, additives, flavorings found in non-organic foods, chemical-laden drinking water, and polluted city air. Off gassing of toxic VOCs (volatile organic compounds) from

building materials, synthetic carpeting, paints, fire retardants and new-car plastics add to the problem. Avoid all weed-killers like Round Up

3. **High-stress sedentary living** with inadequate quality sleep, and inadequate exercise.

Thus, an effective basic optimal health program should include:

1. **A no-sugar, low-carbohydrate, higher protein and medium fat diet** Eliminate all boxed breakfast cereals, soda pop and "electrolyte" sports drinks, all white flour products, all white sugar products, anything containing high-fructose corn syrup, white rice, potato products (chips, hash browns, French fries, tater tots, country fries, mashed, crinkled, boxed). Try to favor organic vegetables and fruits, lots of green salads, <u>grass-fed</u> beef, lamb or veal, non-farmed fish, plenty of black or purple berries. Organic saturated fats from <u>grass-fed</u> animal meats and dairy are necessary for good health. This includes butters (like Kerrygold), organic milk, quality eggs with yolks and some nuts. At least thirty percent of your calories should come from fat. Use Kerrygold butter, olive oil and coconut oil; and avoid all other vegetable

oils, hydrogenated vegetable oils, and margarines. Avoid salami, ham, baloney, processed sandwich meats, hot dogs and carb-containing sausages. Consider avoiding all wheat, rye, and barley (contain gluten). And avoid all soy and corn products (genetically modified). Use only <u>organic</u> grains (free of glyphosate).

2. Make **pure, clean water** your beverage of choice, and add a squeezed lime, or a splash of unsweetened grape juice or pomegranate juice to add some flavor. Simplest and least expensive is to use five-gallon home-delivered Sparkletts or similar quality purified water. These are probably preferable to home installed R.O. (Reverse Osmosis) or other filter systems that require regular testing and maintenance.

   Green and black teas are preferred choices for a hot beverage; coffee too has health benefits, but may also add stresses to the body and be a significant factor if insomnia is a problem. Again, use no sweeteners. Organic whole milk is fine to whiten. Absolutely avoid "non-dairy" creamers.

3. **Exercise**: Critical for distributing oxygen and nutrients to all tissues, including brain. Establish a regular daily (or every other day)

10 – 30 minute routine. Even a thirty-minute brisk walk, using exercise bands, or developing a simple dumb-bell routine (10 lb., 20 lb., 30 lb. weights depending on your strength level) – can add healthy years to your life – and slow brain aging.

4. **Restful sleep** is critically important. Sleep should be on a regular schedule – ideally about eight hours. Avoid all sleep drugs, decrease caffeine beverages after twelve-noon, eat "evening" supper earlier (5 p.m. – 7 p.m.). Late dinners interrupt sleep, increase likelihood of acid reflex (GERD), and will add weight. Avoid late TV news and murder mysteries. Instead consider a warm tub bath, soft music, reading an enjoyable book and meditation before retiring. Add Epsom salts to your tub bath.

5. **Try to avoid all pharmaceutical drugs**, including over-the-counter pain killers, antacids, laxatives and sleeping pills – unless the drug is necessary for life and convincingly prescribed by your physician (such as insulin, glaucoma eye drops, a thyroid medication, or a highly specialized medication for some rare hereditary disorder.)

6. **Intestinal health** is also critically important. Anything less than one to three bowel movements daily is abnormal. Constipation signals poor intestinal health. Using plain unsweetened Kefir or organic yogurt (like Nancy's) and a daily probiotic capsule with 50 billion live bacteria will help restore a healthier balance among the 1,000 plus types of bacteria in your gut. Adequate fruits, vegetables, fiber, and added magnesium are essential for good bowel health. The major cause of constipation and night-time muscle spasms in America is magnesium deficiency.

7. **Stress reduction**. Americans have far too much toxic stress. Discussed earlier, remember to leave time for regular meals, exercise, restful sleep, and spiritual growth. Learn to say NO to burdensome excessive "responsibilities." Add meditation time (like Transcendental Meditation) to your daily program. Leave Sundays for worship, family, friends, fun and rest. Reduce TV, newspapers, magazines, unneeded e-mails, texts, Facebook and tweets.

8. **Avoid toxins** whenever you can – food colorings, preservatives, flavor enhancers (MSG), trans-fats, Agave, high fructose corn syrup, mercury-laced large fish, all forms of tobacco

and smoking, excess alcohol, excess caffeine, pesticides, weed-killers, household chemicals, fabric softeners and air fresheners.

9. Take the following required daily supplements:

- **A <u>simple</u> "complete multi-vitamin-mineral" without iron** (an "Adult 50+" formula). This is a basic, "just to cover the bases" and can be purchased inexpensively. Consider Equate Complete Multivitamin, Adult 50+ at Walmart.

- **Vitamin D3** - 5000 to 10,000 i.u. (international units) daily. Vitamin D3 is critically important to prevent many cancers, colds, and flu, and support cardiovascular and brain health. Don't take less than the 5000 i.u, (for adults) unless you obtain full-body exposure to sunshine for one half hour daily, in which case your body will make over 10,000 i.u. on its own.

- **Magnesium** – 250 to 800 mg daily. Magnesium is important in over 300 cell biochemical reactions, is important to prevent muscle cramps, helps overcome constipation, and supports normal heart rhythm. (Too much Magnesium will cause loose stools. Self regulate what works best for you.)

- **Vitamin K2** (as NK-7) – 100 to 300 micrograms daily

- **Vitamin B12** (sub-lingual, methylcobalamin) – 1,000 to 5,000 micrograms daily, most important for those over age 60.

- **Omega 3, Fish Oil – 2000 mg daily**

- **Boron – 3 mg daily**

And for those "power nutrients" you select to add, these are the recommended adult dosages:

N-Acetyl Cysteine	600 mg
Alpha Lipoic Acid (or R-Lipoic Acid)	300 mg
Green Tea Extract (or drink 3 – 4 cups green or mixed green & black tea daily)	125 mg – 200 mg
Bacopa Monnieri Extract	300 mg

Astaxanthin	4 mg – 10 mg
Resveratrol	25 mg – 100 mg
Grape Seed Extract	200 mg
Curcumin	375 mg – 750 mg
Adaptogens (liquid concentrate)	1/2 dropper sublingual once or twice daily; 3 or 4 daily at times of high stress or illness

All these vitamins and supplements (except where I've provided specific recommendations) can be purchased from vitamin shops, health food stores or your favorite internet sources like Swanson, Puritan, Vitacost – or supermarkets like Wal-Mart, Trader Joe's, Vons, etc.

A final word of wisdom. All of us are unique with different heredity, different stresses, different age and have different histories of diseases, infections, and lifestyles. So when making the new longevity lifestyle choices outlined in this book remember two things:

1. Lifestyle changes and natural plant nutrients (unlike toxic drugs) <u>take time to bring about positive changes</u> – weeks are often required to

start noting positive change – weight loss, higher energy, clearer mind, better memory, elimination of aches and pains, and improved sense of well-being.

2. The right choices of foods and nutrients will make you feel better, not worse. Listen to your body and adjust your program accordingly.

A word to the wise: <u>generally</u>, avoid purchasing any health supplements advertised on television, and especially those offering a "free bottle." Regarding the internet, there are some good products and a few good doctors dispensing advice. But avoid all promotions with the words "Miracle," Magic," "Amazing Breakthrough," "Ultra," "Exclusive," "Fountain of Youth," "Ultimate," "Super Effective," and the likes. There are no magic bullets and never will be. The human body is much, much too complex for such simplistic over-hyped, and usually phony remedies. <u>Trust the basics.</u>

Seventeen

Your Personal Living Healthier Longer Program - Summary

I t's now time to put together your own personalized Living Healthier Longer Program. This is simple, and will effectively move you toward your goal.

1. <u>Follow the dietary and lifestyle changes detailed in Chapter 16</u> Changing habits takes time, so be patient. By weekly re-reading that chapter, you can gradually incorporate all – or most – into your lifestyle.

2. <u>Add the seven basic nutritional supplements listed:</u>

- An inexpensive complete Multi-Vitamin-Mineral, one-a-day type caplet, "to cover the bases." (Adult 50+ formula with no iron).

- Magnesium – 250 mg – 400 mg once or twice daily

- Vitamin D3 – 5000 – 10,000 i.u. daily

- Vitamin K2 (as NK-7) – 100 – 300 mcg daily

- Vitamin B-12 (methylcobolamin) sublingual – 1000 mcg – 5000 mcg daily

- Omega Fish Oil – 2000 mg daily

- Boron – 3 mg daily

3. <u>Review the Power Nutrient Chapters</u> (or the summary of the nutrients in Chapter 14 and dosed in Chapter 16) and select those that offer benefits best suited to your health challenges, or health interests. (All supplements are best taken with a meal).

With these three steps you've put together a premium personal Living Healthier Longer Program and uniquely taken control of your own health: And you're practicing the basics to improve health quality, slow or reverse the aging process, protect DNA telomeres, and positively control thousands of DNA genes that enhance health and longevity.

A final word about this book. It is not a quick-read novel. There is a wealth of health-giving information. So go back and re-read it, underlining issues that are meaningful to you. I am convinced that making these precepts, plans, and products part of your life can easily add ten to thirty years to your life. Practice "Living Healthier Longer" – and you will. This is all about YOU taking charge of your own health !

Let's conclude this book with a few thoughts about the age old practice of Fasting.

Eighteen

What About Fasting?

Fasting has been around for thousands of years. And no, it is not a form of self-abuse, though folks lined up for their third dessert at a Vegas casino buffet might think so.

Fasting, between animal kills, was a normal part of human existence during Paleolithic times.

My belief is that our bodies stay healthiest when we will practice some form of regular fasting.

The only challenge is when, how often, how long, and how to fit it into our busy family and social schedules.

Many religious faiths prescribe regular fasting for self-discipline, spiritual growth, and to break the "sinful habit" of gluttony.

Yogic practice of healing dates back thousands of years. Paramahansa Yogananda claimed, "Fasting is a natural method of healing." And early Western thinkers from Hippocrates to Plato to Socrates all praised the health benefits of fasting. They recognized a revitalizing and rejuvenating power seen with fasting. Many viewed fasting as "the physician within" that could heal and rebalance body energy.

It is worth noting that both animals and humans stop eating and don't want to eat, when we are sick. This decreases stress and allows the body energy to deal with the illness.

Fasting allows the gut to rest and the body to rebalance itself. And it allows the mind to sharpen. I suggest you try the following: One morning after a normal night's sleep, eat no breakfast and drink only pure water until 1:00 PM. No coffee or other stimulant. Your "hunger habit" will make you want to eat, but don't give in. About 11:00 AM or so, you will notice a wonderful clarity of mind setting in.

What's exciting is the scientific support that fasting is now receiving. Most impressive for me is the study done by British physician, Dr. Michael Mosley. Dr. Mosley has found the best way I know to make fasting simple and essentially painless. Total fasting for say three days, - is not easy, takes strong will power, and can result in headaches and fatigue. But Dr. Mosley's technique of two days a week partial fasting is simple, easy to adapt to, and works wonders to improve health. The 5-2 formula works as follows:

I do the "partial fast" on Monday and Thursday (consuming 600 calories for men, 500 calories for women) and eating your regular diet the other 5 days. For exact details and nice color pictures of the meals, get a copy of Dr. Mosley's book, "The Fast Diet" (e.g. Amazon Books). It's become an international best seller!

For my "longevity" interest, a very important finding by Dr. Mosely was that the 5-2 Fast diet, significantly lowered Insulin Growth Factor-1 (IGF-1). Many doctors mistakenly suggest that we should elevate IGF-1. That's, in fact, what HGH (Human Growth Hormone) does.

But good studies indicate that elevation of IGF-1 increases cell growth and increases the incidence of many cancers! Exactly what you don't want. So, avoid all products or clinic injections that elevate HGH, and IGF-1.

Fasting can be fun and you can test its health benefits yourself.

And yes, it will help you achieve your ideal weight while improving your health.

As traditional allopathic medicine evolves toward Anti-Aging holistic medicine, fasting will find its place as an invaluable aid to self-healing and Living Healthier Longer.

Bibliography

1. Joseph JA, Shukitt-Hale B, Lau FC. "Fruit poly-phenols and their effects on neuronal signaling and behavior in senescence." *Ann N Y Acad Sci 2007 Apr;1100:470-85.*

2. Shukitt-Hale B, Lau FC, Joseph JA. "Berry fruit supplementation and the aging brain." *J Agric Food Chem 2008 Feb 13;56(3):636-41. Epub 2008 Jan 23.*

3. Joseph JA, Shukitt-Hale B, Casadesus G. "Reversing the deleterious effects of aging on neuronal communication and behavior: benefi-cial properties of fruit polyphenolic compounds." *Am J Clin Nutr. 2005 Jan;81(1 Suppl):313S-316S.*

4. Willis LM, Shukitt-Hale B, Joseph JA. "Recent advances in berry supplementation and age-related cognitive decline." *Curr Opin Clin Nutr Metab Care. 209 Jan;12(1):91-4.*

5. Erlund I, et al. "Favorable effects of berry consumption on platelet function, blood pressure, and HDL cholesterol." *Am J Clin Nutr. 2008 Feb 87, No.(2):323-331.*

6. Phytonutrient Graphics. "Oxygen radical absorbance capacity comparisons."

7. Hildalgo MA, Jara E, Ojedal, Hancke JL, Burgos RA, "Effect of Aristotelia chilensis (Maqui) on inflammation response." *Laboratory of Molecular Pharmacology, Universidad Austral de Chile.*

8. Kawahara M, "Effects of aluminum on the nervous system and its possible link with neurodegenerative diseases." *J Alzheimers Dis.* 2005 Nov;8(2):171-82.

9. Miranda-Rottmann S, Aspillaga AA, Perez DD, Vasquez L, Martinez AL, Leighton F, "Juice and phenolic fractions of the berry Aristotelia chilensis inhibit LDL, oxidation in vitro and protect human endothelial cells against

oxidative stress." *Agric Food Chem. 2002 Dec 18:50(26):7542-7*

10. Franco R, Schoneveld OJ, Pappa A, Panaviotidis MI. "The central role of glutathione in the pathophysiology of human disease." *Arch Physiol Biochem. 2007 Oct-Dec;113(4-5):234-58.*

11. Miquel J, Ferrandiz ML, De Juan E, Sevila I, Martinez M. "N-acetylcysteine protects against age-related decline of oxidative phosphorylation in liver mitochondria." *Eur J Pharmacol.* 1995 Mar 16;292(3-4):333.5.

12. Navarro A, Boveris A. "The mitochondrial energy transduction system and the aging process." *Am J Physiol Cell Physiol.* 2007 Feb;292(2):C670-86. Epub 2006 Oct 4.

13. "The Book of Tea" 2005, Flammarion Publishers

14. Choi YT. et al. "The green tea polyphenol epigallocatechin gallate attenutates beta-amyloid-induced neurotoxicity in cultured hippocampal neurons." *Life Sci.* 2001 Dec 21;70(5):603-14.

15. Bettuzzi S. et al. A. "Chemo prevention of human prostate cancer by oral administration of

green tea catechins in volunteers with high-grade prostate intraepithelial neoplasia: a preliminary report from a one-year proof-of-principle study." *Cancer Res.* 2006 Jan 15;66(2):1234-40.

16. Kurivama S, et al. "Green tea consumption and mortality due to cardiovascular disease, cancer and all causes in Japan: the Ohsaki study. "*JAMA.* 2006 Sept 13;296(10):1255-65.

17. Seely D, Mills EJ, Wu P, Verma S, Guyatt GH. "The effects of green tea consumption on incidence of breast cancer and recurrence of breast cancer: a systematic review and meta-analysis." *Integr Cancer Ther.* 2005 June;4(2):144-55.

18. Wu CH, et al. "Epidemiological evidence of increased bone mineral density in habitual tea drinkers." *Arch Intern Med.* 2002 May 13;162(9):1001-6.

19. Geleijnse, JM, et al. "Inverse association of tea and flavonoid intakes with incident myocardial infarction: the Rotterdam Study." *Am J Clin Nutr.* 2002 May;75(5):880-6.

20. Roodenrys S, et al. "Chronic effects of Brahmi (Bacopa monnieri) on human memory." *Neuropsychopharmacology.* 2002 Aug;27(2):279-81.

21. Anbaraski K, Vani G, Devi CS. "Protective effects of bacoside A on cigarette smoking-induced brain mitochondrial dysfunction in rats." *J Environ Pathol Toxicol Oncol.* 2005; 24(3):225-34.

22. Bhattacharya SK, Bhattacharya A, Kumar A, Ghosal S. "Antioxidant activity of Bacopa monniera in rat frontal cortex, striatum and hippocampus." *Phytother Res.* 2000 May;14(3):174-9.

23. Stough C. et al. "The chronic effects of an extract of Bacopa monniera (Brahmi) on cognitive function in healthy human subjects." *Psychopharmacology (Berl).* 2001 Aug;156(4):481-4.

24. Russo A, et al. "Free radical scavenging capacity and protective effect of Bacopa monniera L. on DNA damage." *Phytother Res.* 2003 Sep;17(8):870-5.

25. Viji V, Helen A. "Inhibition of lipoxygenases and cyclooxygenase-2 enzymes by extracts

isolated from Bacopa monniera (L.) Wettst." *J Ethnopharmacol.* 2008 Jul23;118(2):305-11.

26. Stough C. et al. "Examining the nootropic effects of a special extract of Bacopa monniera on human cognitive functioning: 90 day double-blind placebo-controlled randomized trial." *Phytother Res.* 2008 Dec;22(12):1629-34.

27. Calabrese C., et al. "Effects of a standardized Bocopa monnieri extract on cognitive performance, anxiety, and depression in the elderly: a randomized, double-blind, placebo-controlled trial." *J Altern Complement Med.* 2008 Jul;14(6):707-13.

28. Jyoti A, Sharma D. "Neuroprotective role of Bacopa monniera extract against aluminum-induced oxidative stress in the hippocampus of rat brain." *Neurotoxicology.* 2006 Jul;27(4):451-7.

29. Limpeanchob N., et al. "Neuroprotective effects of Bacopa monnieri on beta-amyloid-induced cell death in primary cortical culture." *J Ethnopharmacol.* 2008 Oct 30;120(1):112-7.

30. Samiulla DS, Prashanth D, Amit A. "Mast cell stabilizing activity of Bacopa monnieri." *Fitoterapia.* 2001 Mar;72(3):284-5.

31. Higuera-Ciapara I, Felix-Valenzuela L, Goycoolea FM. "Astaxanthin: a review of its chemistry and applications." *Crit Rev Food Sci Nutr.* 2006;46(2):185-96.

32. Hussein G., et al. "Axtaxanthin, a carotenoid with potential in human health and nutrition." *J Na Prod.* 2006 Mar;69(3):443-9.

33. Hussein G., et al. "Antihypertensive and neuroprotective effects of axtaxanthin in experimental animals." *Bio Pharm Bull.* 2005 Jan;28(1):47-52.

34. Mason RP., et al. "Rofecoxib increases susceptibility of human LDL and membrane lipids to oxidative damage: a mechanism of cardiotoxicity." *J Cardiovasc Pharmacol.* 2006;47 Suppl 1:S7-14.

35. Chew BP, Park JS. "Carotenoid action on the immune response." *J Nutr.* 2004 Jan;134(1): 257S-261S.

36. Tanaka T., et al. "Chemoprevention of mouse urinary bladder carcinogenesis by the naturally occurring carotenoid astaxanthin." *Carcinogenesis* 1994 Jan;15(1):15-9.

37. Chew BP., et al. "A comparison of the anticancer activities of dietary beta-carotene, canthaxanthin and astaxanthin in mice in vivo." *Anticancer Res.* 1999 Ma-Jun;19(3A):1849-53.

38. Orallo F. "Trans-resveratrol: a magical elixir of eternal youth?" *Curr Med Chem.* 2008;15(19): 1887-98.

39. Nicholson SK, Tucker GA, Brameld JM. "Effects of dietary polyphenols on gene expression in human vascular endothelial cells." *Proc Nutr Soc.* 2008 Feb;67(1):42-7.

40. Brito PM., et al. "Resveratrol affords protection against peroxynitrite-mediated endothelial cell death: A role for intracellular glutathione." *Chem Biol Interact.* 2006 Dec 15;164(3):157-66.

41. Pallas M., et al. "Resveratrol and neurodegenerative diseases: activation of SIRT1 as the potential pathway towards neuroprotection." *Curr Neurovasc Res.* 2009 Feb;6(1):70-81.

42. Karuppagounder SS., et al. "Dietary supplementation with resveratrol reduces plaque pathology in a transgenic model of Alzheimer's disease." *Neurochem Int.* 2009 Feb;54(2):111-8.

43. Park YM, Febbraio M, Silverstein R. "CD36 modulates migration of mouse and human macrophages in response to oxidized LDL and may contribute to macrophage trapping in the arterial intima." *J Clin Invest.* 2009 Jan 5;119(1):136-145.

44. Curtiss, LK. "Reversing Atherosclerosis?" *NEJM.* March 12, 2009.

45. Sivaprakasapillai B., et al. "Effects of grape seed extract on blood pressure in subjects with the metabolic syndrome." *Metab Clin Exp.*" 2009.

46. Editorial. "The 1998 Nobel prize in Medicine: clinical implications." *Vasc Med.* 1999 (2):57-60.

47. Edirisinghe I., et al. "Mechanism of the endothelium-dependent relaxation evoked by a grape seed extract." *Clin Sci* 2008;114:331-337.

48. Del Bas JM., et al. "Grape seed procyanidins improve atherosclerotic risk index and induce liver CLYP7A1 and SHP expression in healthy rats." *FASEB J.* 2005 Mar;19(3):479-81.

49. Bagchi D., et al. "Molecular mechanisms of cardioprotection by a novel grape seed

proanthocyanidin extract." *Mutat Res.* 2003 Feb-Mar;523-524:87-97.

50. Del Bas JM., et al. "Dietary procyanidins lower triglyceride levels signaling through the nuclear receptor small heterodimer partner." *Mol Nutr Food Res.* 2008 Oct;52(10):1172-81.

51. Wang J., et al. "Grape-derived polyphenolics prevent Abeta oligomerization and attenuate cognitive deterioration in a mouse model of Alzheimer's disease." *J Neurosci.* 2008 Jun 18;28(25):6388-92.

52. Wang J., et al. "Grape-derived polyphenolics prevent Abeta oligomerization and attenuate cognitive deterioration in a mouse model of Alzheimer's disease." *J Neurosci.* 2008 Jun 18;28(25):6388-92.

53. Ono K., et al. "Effects of grape seed-derived polyphenols on amyloid beta-protein self-assembly and cytotoxicity." *J Biol Chem.* 2008 Nov 21;283(47):32176-87.

54. Kaur M, Mandair R, Agarwal R, Agarwal C. "Grape seed extract induces cell cycle arrest

and apoptosis in human colon carcinoma cells." *Nurt Cancer* 2008;60 Suppl 1:2-11.

55. Aggarwal BB., et al. "Curcumin: the Indian solid gold." *Adv Exp Med Biol.* 2007;595:1-75.

56. Yang F., et al. "Curcumin inhibits formation of amyloid beta oligomers and fibrils, binds plaques, and reduces amyloid in vivo." *J Biol Chem.* 2005 Feb 18;280(7):5892-901.

57. Hatcher H., et al. "Curcumin: from ancient medicine to current clinical trials." *Cell Mol Life Sci.* 2008 Jun;65(11):1631-52.

58. Houska R., "If you were to stretch all the body's blood vessels end to end..." *Mad Sci Net.* 1999 Jan 10;19:08:17.

59. Schechezhin AK, Zinkovich VI, and Galanova LK, "Eleutherococcus prephylaxis of influenza, hypertension and heart ischemia of Auto VAZ drivers." *New Data on Eleutherococcus and Other Adaptogens,* The Far Eastern Scientific Center, Russian Academy of Sciences, Vladivostok (1981)

Disclaimer Regarding
Information in this Book

This book makes no claims to diagnose, treat, or cure any classified disease.

Because good health implies the absence of recognized diseases, and because the best scientific studies of health and nutrition relate their studies to known diseases, these worlds understandably intersect and inter-relate.

But the information in this book is for educational purposes only so that its readers can more intelligently make the food, supplement, and lifestyle choices to improve their health and quality of life.

The FDA does not evaluate food supplements, nor has it evaluated the information in this book. All serious health conditions should be evaluated and managed by a competent health practitioner. Neither the author, nor the publisher of this book are herein dispensing medical diagnosis or treatment; nor do we assume responsibility for readers who choose to treat themselves.

46014999R10080

Made in the USA
San Bernardino, CA
24 February 2017